The Medicare Part D Drug Program

Making the Most of the Benefit

Jack E. Fincham, PhD, RPh

A.W. Jowdy Professor of Pharmacy Care
Adjunct Professor of Public Health
The University of Georgia
College of Pharmacy
Athens, GA

JONES AND BARTLETT F
Sudbury, Massachuset
BOSTON   TORONTO   LONDON

D1057757

World Headquarters
Jones and Bartlett Publishers
40 Tall Pine Drive
Sudbury, MA 01776
978-443-5000
info@jbpub.com
www.jbpub.com

Jones and Bartlett Publishers
Canada
6339 Ormindale Way
Mississauga, Ontario L5V
1J2
CANADA

Jones and Bartlett Publishers
International
Barb House, Barb Mews
London W6 7PA
UK

Jones and Bartlett's books and products are available through most bookstores and online book-sellers. To contact Jones and Bartlett Publishers directly, call 800-832-0034, fax 978-443-8000, or visit our website, www.jbpub.com.

Substantial discounts on bulk quantities of Jones and Bartlett's publications are available to corporations, professional associations, and other qualified organizations. For details and specific discount information, contact the special sales department at Jones and Bartlett via the above contact information or send an email to specialsales@jbpub.com.

Production Credits
Executive Editor: Dave Cella
Editorial Assistant: Lisa Gordon
Production Director: Amy Rose
Associate Production Editor: Daniel Stone
Associate Marketing Manager: Jen Bengtson
Manufacturing Buyer: Amy Bacus
Cover Design: Kristin Ohlin
Cover Photo Credits: © Purestock/Getty Images (top image of cover)
                     © Photos.com (bottom image of cover)
Composition: Maggie Dana/Pageworks
Printing and Binding: Malloy, Inc.
Cover Printing: Malloy, Inc.

Library of Congress Cataloging-in-Publication Data
Fincham, Jack E.
    The Medicare part D drug program : making the most of the benefit / Jack Fincham.
      p. cm.
    ISBN-13: 978-0-7637-4967-5
    ISBN-10: 0-7637-4967-2
    1. United States. Medicare Prescription Drug, Improvement, and Modernization Act of 2003. 2. Older people—Pharmaceutical assistance—United States. 3. Insurance, Pharmaceutical services—United States. 4. Medicare. I. Title.
    RA412.3.F56 2007
    368.38'200973—dc22   2006032664
    6048

This publication is designed to provide accurate and authoritative information in regard to the subject matter covered. It is sold with the understanding that the publisher is not engaged in rendering legal, accounting, or other professional service. If legal advice or other expert assistance is required, the service of a competent professional person should be sought.

Printed in the United States of America

To Busby Berkley, thank you for all your support, encouragement, and friendship. Your thoughtful comments throughout the writing of this text have been invaluable.

Contents

Contents

Chapter 10. Getting Your Drugs and Drug Taking in Order   *123*

Chapter 11. Summary and Next Steps   *133*

The passage of the Medicare Prescription Drug, Improvement, and Modernization Act (MMA) was monumental legislation when passed in 2003 for the American public. For the first time, for those greater than age 65 and other specific sectors of the population, a benefit (Medicare Part D) was made available to partially pay for the costs of prescription medications. However, the path traveled from passage in 2003 to enactment in January of 2006, and ultimately delivering the benefit to beneficiaries, has been a road embedded with enrollment processes not easily navigated, confusing directions, perplexing terminology (to the public and healthcare providers alike), misunderstood benefits, and a sea of acronyms. While the journey itself may have proven confusing for those that embarked upon it, it is the final destination here that remains the focus—prescription coverage for those who are in need of it.

The author begins with an overview of the alphabet soup of other Medicare Insurance benefits that have come before (A, B, and C) while focusing on the new prescription benefit—Medicare Part D, beginning with how the program works, including the famed "donut hole" or gap in coverage, and if one is even eligible to enroll in the program. Readers must remember that there are limits to what is covered and how much is covered annually. Furthermore, readers are encouraged to use the resources provided in the ensuing chapters to determine calculated medication spending for a given year.

Dr. Fincham helps guide beneficiaries through the process of choosing an insurance plan (recognizing that one does not simply sign up for the benefit but also needs to pick an insurance provider to administer the prescription drug plan) as well as how to determine which medications are covered under the insurance plan's "formulary," noting that not all medications are covered. The formulary can be thought of as a wine list of medications. While you may desire (or your physician may desire for you) a specific red wine, the wine list made available to you by your selected insurance provider of the prescription drug plan may contain many red wines but not the specific one desired (e.g., prescribed). Hence, some adjustment in therapy or an intervention by your physician will be necessary to make sure you obtain a medication that is appropriate for you from your plan at the pharmacy. Note, it is the plan that determines what medications are available to the beneficiary, not the pharmacy. Thus, communication among patients, physicians, plan administrators, and pharmacists is paramount to ensure smooth transactions.

While the highlight of the Medicare Part D Program is payment for prescription medications for beneficiaries, an important player in helping patients achieve optimal outcomes from their medication therapies is the pharmacist. Without a conductor to lead the orchestra (e.g., a pharmacist), the musicians (e.g., multiple prescribers of medications), while well intentioned, may not play together harmoniously. Likewise, the notes on the pages (e.g., prescriptions) may be overlooked or misinterpreted, not knowing the full score of music to be played or played previously (e.g., current and previous medications used). Think of the pharmacist as a conductor of appropriate medication use—helping you or a loved one achieve the appropriate outcomes from the intended therapy prescribed, while avoiding the potentially ill effects of some medications, and intervening when necessary with your physician. One cautionary caveat is that not using the same conductor can lead to miscommunication and less than optimal care and outcomes. Thus, take care to select one pharmacist you trust, as you would your physician.

The concluding chapters provide the reader with additional tools to assist them or others with their medication use (i.e., medication therapy management services, preventive services, screening tests, health promotion, and tips to improve taking medications). In the final chapter, Dr. Fincham alludes to anticipated changes to the Medicare Part D benefit in 2007 and beyond. Recognizing that this is a new benefit, originally estimated to cost the government (tax payers) around $43 billion in the first year alone (though estimates put the price tag at $30 billion in the inaugural year), there will be ongoing changes to this program. Some changes will be viewed positively and some negatively. Whether a direct beneficiary now, a future beneficiary, or assisting others with this benefit (including healthcare providers), this book is surely one that should not be far from the reader's grasp in trying to understand and maximize this benefit.

George E. MacKinnon III, PhD, RPh
Vice President of Academic Affairs
American Association of Colleges of Pharmacy

This book will help you use the new Medicare Part D drug benefit to your best advantage. The coverage of prescription drugs in the Medicare program is a major change in the insurance available for health care for seniors. Since 1965, when Medicare was enacted, seniors have faced many dilemmas when choosing to purchase prescription drugs. Up until now, you had to pay for drugs on your own or through other insurance policies. This coverage lag of 40 years in needed coverage for medications has led to severe hardships for many. Now, you can receive help with the cost of your prescription drugs in the new Medicare Part D program. The reason I wrote this book is to help you gain as much as you can through this new Medicare option. Some of you who are eligible have been or will be assigned a Part D plan due to your being eligible for both Medicare and Medicaid. The vast majority must sign up in a defined period of time. If you do not have other coverage for drugs, failure to sign up when you have the window of opportunity will cost you money and I want you to avoid this at all costs! If you have drug coverage that is as good as or better than is available with Medicare Part D, you can keep your current coverage and not sign up for Medicare Part D.

I want you to be able to make choices in this program that will benefit you or those for whom you provide care. Many aspects of this program are hard to understand. Formularies, provider status, co-payments, deductibles, and petitions for service are several confusing elements of Medicare Part D. My goal is to simplify the components of this benefit. You can then best prepare to use Medicare Part D for your advantage. The Part D program will undoubtedly change in the coming months and subsequent years. The more you can do to educate yourself about the benefit now will help you in the coming months and beyond.

You may be eligible for extra coverage under Medicare Part D. I want you to know how to determine if you can receive extra benefits. Also, you will want to choose a program that allows you to continue to take the drugs you are taking now at the lowest cost available. This will take some time to figure out, but you can do this easily. You may need to have someone help you, but the extra effort at the start of your seeking a plan will help you later on. If you can use a computer and access the

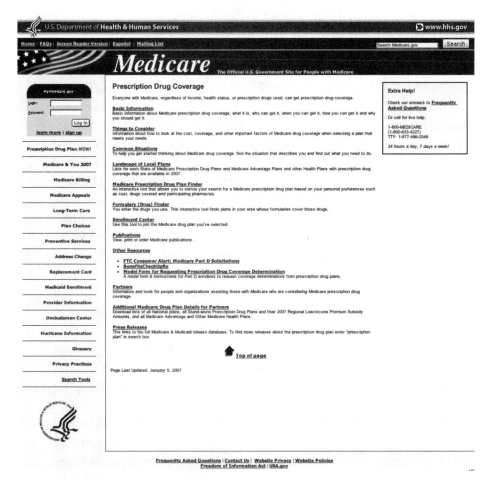

Prescription Drug Coverage, PDP Main Page
Source: http://www.medicare.gov.pdphome.asp

www.mymedicare.gov Web site and the Web sites for the various Prescription Drug Plans (www.medicare.gov/pdphome.asp) and Medicare Advantage plans (www.medicare.gov/Choices/Advantage.asp) you will be in a much better position to help yourself make the very best decisions that you can. If you have a friend or faculty member that can use a computer, this will be a big help to you in the decision making process.

There are countless sources of Part D information available for your use. Some of these "informational sources" might have a motive to sell you something. This book is not written with that intent. Use this book and the

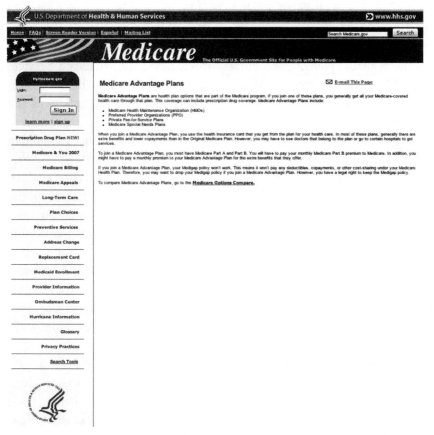

Prescription Drug Coverage, Medicare Advantage Main Page
Source: http://www.medicare.gov./Choices/Advantage.asp

references provided to start making the most of Medicare Part D now. Learn as much as you can so you can make the right choices. Help save yourself time and money with benefits to your health.

I want to help you make the best choices for your particular needs. These choices begin with whether to sign up or not. Next you must decide which program to sign up for. Other questions are important for you to consider: Which pharmacies will continue to provide the drugs I need? What drugs are covered? How to obtain your medications when you are told some of your drugs are not covered. This might be a very good time for you to look at the drugs you take and see if any of them can be eliminated. Work with your doctors and pharmacist to help identify drugs that you perhaps do not need to take. This will save you time and be of benefit to your health at the same time. Not all pharmacies will be able to fill your prescriptions in some of the available plans. The Centers for Medicare and Medicaid Services (CMS) have useful websites that can help you understand the differences between plans. The www.medicare.gov Web site shows several items you can click on to find out more information.

There are examples throughout the book and the reference material in the back of the book will take you step by step through the Medicare Part D plan. These segments will help you understand the benefit; choose which one is right for you, how you can obtain additional financial help if you are eligible, and determine which of your drugs are covered. You may not need to sign up for Medicare Part D if you have coverage for drugs from insurance from your former employer. What if your former employer changes your retiree medical insurance and drops or decreases prescription coverage? We will explore what to do if your insurance from your former employer changes and you then no longer have coverage. You will also learn how to go about switching plans if you find out that another option might be better for you.

You may ask several questions about the pharmacy to use for your prescription needs. Can you as an individual really make the necessary decisions? How bad a choice can you make? Is it automatically something more than you can handle? What if you do nothing? Does it matter what pharmacy you use to fill your prescriptions? What is in-network and what is out-of-network? Will you have to use mail order pharmacies? You may have a "Medigap" drug policy and wonder if you need to apply for Medicare Part D. Each of these questions will be answered. I have learned about this plan by studying it and helping people like you find the best plan for them. I will help you make the best choice for a Medicare Part D prescription drug plan.

Jack Fincham

CHAPTER 1

The Medicare Part D Program

What Is Medicare?

Medicare is the insurance program that is available to you when you reach retirement age. If you are not already getting retirement benefits, you should contact the Social Security Administration about three months before you reach age 65 to sign up for Medicare. You can sign up for Medicare even if you do not plan to retire at age 65. Once you are enrolled in Medicare, you will receive your red, white, and blue Medicare card showing whether you have Part A, Part B, or both.

Medicare Part A

The following quote is from the Social Security Administration website (www.ssa.gov):

> Keep your card in a safe place so you will have it when you need it. If your card is ever lost or stolen, you can *apply for a replacement card* on the Internet at www.socialsecurity.gov or call Social Security's toll-free number. You will also receive a *Medicare & You* (Publication No. CMS-10050) handbook that describes your Medicare benefits and Medicare plan choices.

Medicare Part A coverage will pay for your hospital bills and some of your doctor's charges as well.

Medicare Part B

Again from the www.ssa.gov website, the following is the information about receiving Medicare Part B benefits:

> "When you first become eligible for hospital insurance (Part A), you have a seven-month period (your initial enrollment period) in which to sign up for medical insurance (Part B). A delay on your part will cause a delay in coverage and result in higher premiums. If you are eligible at age 65, your initial enrollment period begins three months before your 65th birthday, including the month you turn age 65 and ending three months after that birthday. If you are eligible for Medicare based on disability or permanent kidney failure, your initial enrollment period depends on the date your disability or treatment began."

New Program in Medicare

The Medicare Prescription Drug, Improvement, and Modernization Act became law on December 8, 2003. More commonly known as the Medicare Modernization Act (MMA), this law will affect how you can obtain additional help in the Medicare program.

What is this new program in Medicare? There is now a part of Medicare insurance that *can help pay for some or a large portion of your prescription costs*. This program is Medicare Part D. This is a new program that started on January 1, 2006. You are not automatically enrolled in Medicare Part D, and you must enroll during a period of time for the best rates. If you do not, you will be assessed a penalty charge per month that will continue each month even if you have enrolled.

There are some individuals covered by Medicare that will automatically be assigned to a Medicare Part D Plan. This is due to their financial circumstances. Unless you are in this category, you will need to pay an insurance premium monthly, and pay a portion of the cost of your drugs. This amount you pay will vary in coverage as you progress through the year and buy your drugs throughout the year.

Caution About Scam Artists

You should be extra cautious about scam artists that may try to take advantage of you! If someone tries to sell you insurance and asks for bank information, they are not to be trusted. Likewise, if someone claims that you can obtain a new Medicare insurance card for an amount of money, they too are trying to take advantage of you. So, please be cautious about those from whom you seek information or insurance coverage.

Nowhere are people immune from these scams. Since the start of the program in January 2006 there have been complaints from seniors about telephone contacts from individuals. These individuals represent themselves as agents for Medicare Part D insurance companies. Callers have represented themselves as representing non-existent but legitimate sounding groups. The offer is to help seniors with the difficult Medicare Part D program. The callers then ask for money or credit card numbers to provide service to individuals. It is important that you realize that no legitimate Medicare Part D Plan will ask for money or credit card information over the phone.

Complaints About Medicare Part D

Things will not always go okay with any governmental program, including Medicare Part D. There have been around 2.2 complaints per 1,000 Medicare beneficiaries enrolled in the new prescription drug plans. Many of the complaints have dealt with issues pertaining to enrolling or disenrolling in plans. Also, the costs of co-payments with drugs and access to drugs have been issues. If you suspect that you are being treated unfairly or are the target of a scam artist, you can register a complaint. Often we feel reluctant to do something like complain. In this case, please do. It will help not only you but save others a similar problem as well. Complaints of possible fraud, waste, and abuse can be reported to the United States Office of Inspector General's (OIG) Hotline in several ways. You can call toll-free phone: 1-800-HHS-TIPS (1-800-447-8477). The line is operated from 8:00 am–5:30 pm, Eastern Time, Monday-Friday. You can also send a fax to 1-800-223-8164 (10 pages or less) or email your complaint to hhstips@oig.hhs.gov. Furthermore, you can send a letter via mail to:

HHS TIPS Hotline
P.O. Box 23489
Washington, DC 20026

You can also access the OIG Hotline guide for filing a complaint by going to the OIG Website at www.oig.hhs.gov/hotline.html. A copy of this web site has been included later in the chapter and see Figure 1–1 for a depiction of the OIG web site.

So How Can I Benefit from Medicare Part D?

Medicare Part D is the part of Medicare health insurance that helps pay some of your prescription drug costs.

Medicare insurance is the government program that provides health insurance for seniors once you reach age 65 years. Medicare Part D is the segment of Medicare that now pays for some of your prescription drug costs. Please see Table 1–1 for a listing of the various Medicare programs and what items the Medicare "Part" will cover for you.

When Did Medicare Part D Start?

Medicare Part D began on January 1, 2006. This program is provided by companies that you must sign up with. These companies can be stand alone units (prescription drug plans), or part of a Medicare Advantage plan (a managed care plan that provides several types of coverage options). Unlike

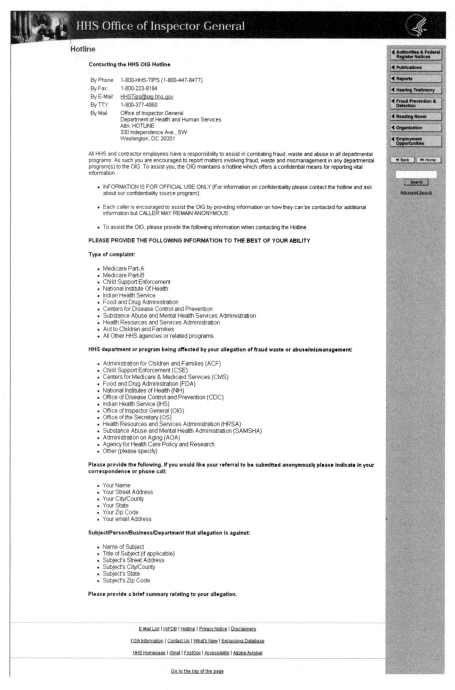

Figure 1–1   HHS Office of Inspector General, Hotline
Source: http://oig.hhs.gov/hotline.html

Table 1–1 Medicare Insurance Programs			
Medicare component (Part)	What does it cover?	What type of services are included?	Do you need to sign up for the plan?
Part A	Hospital Insurance	Inpatient hospital services, skilled nursing facilities, home care.	Eligible at age 65 years. Payroll taxes finance the plan so you pay no premiums
Part B	Supplemental Medical Insurance	Physician and other health care provider office visits, outpatient services, drugs administered in an outpatient clinic.	Pay by premiums which vary per month, and the rates are raised each year. You must sign up for Part B Medicare.
Medicare Advantage	Medicare Advantage (managed care) Formerly Medicare Choice, or Medicare Part C	Medicare Parts A, B, and D provided through a private health plan such as a managed care organization (HMO).	You sign up for this plan and it is paid for by a combination of payroll taxes and premiums.
Part D	Prescription Drug Insurance	Outpatient prescription drugs such as those purchased in a community pharmacy or from an outpatient hospital pharmacy.	Premiums vary depending upon which plan you choose. You must sign up for coverage.

It is important to note that you must sign up for Medicare Part D, you are not automatically enrolled.

Medicare Part A, you must sign up for Medicare Part D—you are not automatically enrolled.

What Pharmacies Can I Use to Obtain My Prescriptions?

In order to provide as much coverage as possible, many pharmacies can fill your prescriptions under this benefit. However, not all pharmacies may be in the network (listing of pharmacies eligible to be used in your prescription plan), so you may not be able to use your normal pharmacy. This is something that you should check on before you sign up for a plan. Many pharmacies belong to many networks and thus can fill your prescriptions; others may not be able to.

Find out if your regular pharmacy is part of the network of eligible pharmacies in your Medicare Part D plan.

Are Your Drugs Covered?

This is really important for you to spend time considering. The issue is that all the drugs that you take now may not be covered in a plan that you might choose. This means that you will have to pay for the drug out of your own pocket if you choose a particular plan without coverage for your drug. A recent study conducted by the Kaiser Family Foundation concluded that on average, 80% of a listing of commonly used drugs was covered under most plans participating in Medicare Part D (2). No plan covered all the drugs, and the range of coverage was from 64-97% (1). Most plans operate with what is termed a tiered coverage scheme. The tiers are differing types of drugs that you will pay different amounts of co-payments or cost-sharing amounts. See Table 1–2 for an example of how tiers in a formulary work.

Know which of your drugs are available as generic substitutes and have your pharmacist help you with this. This is a key way to save yourself money with this program.

What About Other Assistance Programs?

There are several pharmaceutical company assistance programs that can help you with coverage for your drugs when the gap in your insurance comes into play. These programs and information about them can be found at the following internet sites:

- A program by Schering-Plough Pharmaceuticals: www.schering-plough.com; 1-800-521-7157

The issue is that all the drugs you take now may not be covered in a plan you might choose. This means you will have to pay for the drug out of your own pocket if you choose a particular plan without coverage for your drug.

The Medicare Part D Program

Table 1–2	An Example of a Tiered Arrangement For a Type of Drug	
Tier	Drugs covered	Amount to pay
First tier	A generically available drug (generic)	$5.00
Second tier	A preferred brandname drug	$25.00
Third tier	A non-preferred brand drug	$60.00

- Partnership for prescription assistance: www.pparx.org; 1-888-4PPA-NOW
- A listing of various state pharmaceutical assistance programs and how they can be contacted can be found at the following website sponsored by the National Association of Chain Drugstores: http://www.nacds.org/wmspage.cfm?parm1=4568

Some of you may also have a coverage policy from your previous employer that still covers your prescription drugs after you retire. If this plan is just as good or better than the Medicare Part D Plans, you do not have to sign up for one. You might also have benefits through the United States Veterans Administration (VA). If this is the case, you also do not need to sign up for Medicare Part D.

Signing Up for Medicare Part D

Please know that if you are eligible to sign up for Medicare Part D, you may choose not to sign up for coverage. However, if you do not sign up in the time period you are allowed to do so, you will have to pay an additional amount per month (a 1% penalty) plus the regular amount of the monthly premium. It is also important for you to know that once you sign up for a particular plan, you must stay with this plan for the balance of the year. However, if you are dissatisfied with the plan that you originally signed up for, you can change to a different plan for the next year.

So What Do I Need to Know to Get Started?

There are several key things that you need to know to obtain the most from this benefit. I do not expect that you know the answers to these questions now. However, by the end of the book you will have a better idea of what these issues mean to you.

You should know the answers to the following:

- Know your drugs. What are the drugs that you take and their complete names?
- Know your pharmacist. Will the pharmacy you use be able to continue to take care of your needs?
- Know which of your drugs are available as generic substitutes. Have your pharmacist help you with this. Using as many generics drugs as you can will be a key way to save money with this program.
- Know about how much you will spend for drugs per year. Ask your pharmacist to help you with this.
- Know as much as you can about the Medicare Part D benefit. Do you know how to make this benefit work for you?
- Know what the 'donut hole' gap in coverage means to you and how to make sure that you can diminish its impact on your costs.
- Know who can help you with understanding this program and its components.

Please see the second page United States Federal Trade Commission "Consumer Alert" at the end of this chapter. This alert provides tips for you to employ to keep from being a fraud victim.

References

1. Hoadley J, Hargrave E, Cubanski J, Neuman T. An in-depth examination of formularies and other features of Medicare drug plans, Washington, DC: *The Henry J. Kaiser Family Foundation, Report # 7489*, April, 2006.

CHAPTER 2

How Will This Program Work and How Can I Determine What Is Best For Me?

You will have access to the Medicare Part D benefit through two basic types of plans. These plans differ in scope of coverage and the amount charged for premiums. Careful consideration is necessary when deciding on the plan to choose. Let me start by defining what these two plans are.

Private Prescription Drug Plans (PDPs) (This Material Is Adapted from the www.cms.gov Website)

These free standing plans will provide services on a fee for service basis. This means that you will pay for your medications as you always do until you reach a certain amount that you have paid. This is called a deductible. As you start the coverage with this plan, you will pay for your prescriptions until you reach the amount paid of $265 for 2007. Some of the plans have not required this deductible amount. They have done so to try to get as many people as possible to sign up for the coverage. The trade-off that you have to consider is you may pay a little more for a monthly premium, but you will not have to pay any deductible. You might also have coverage in the so called "donut hole" and have coverage for your drugs throughout the year. It is really important to consider all these facts when you decide on a plan. Also, realize that although you are tied to a plan once you sign up for the balance of the year, you can switch plans for the next year. Therefore a plan that does not meet all your needs one year can be dropped for another plan for the next year.

There are several things that you can decide about the PDPs and the differences between them. Each plan will provide an overview of important information about each PDP: how much the premiums are monthly, what the PDP will pay for and what it covers, and whether the PDP offers a mail service prescription option. In the Medicare website and in their written materials there will be numerous things that you can consider. There are several types of information available for each plan.

The Name of the Organization

This will be the name of the company offering the Medicare drug plan. Some sponsoring organizations may offer more than one Medicare drug plan. There may be names such as Humana PDP Standard, Humana PDP Enhanced, Humana PDP Complete as an example (www.humana-medicare.com/medicare-part-d.asp). I am using Human here as an example. I did not include the company here out of any favoritism.

The Actual Plan Name

The name of the Medicare PDP drug plan, e.g., Humana PDP Standard.

Cost

This is the total amount you would pay the plan each month for your health care and prescription drug coverage. There may be several things to think about with the options here for you to consider:

1. You may pay *no* premium with Full Low Income Subsidy. If you get full extra help from Medicare paying for your prescription drugs, you will not have to pay a premium.
2. Drug Deductible: This is the amount you will pay before the drug plan begins to pay.
3. Zero: This might be a component of a plan you choose, and in this case you do not have to pay anything before the plan begins to pay.
4. Reduced: You pay less than $265 before the plan begins to pay.
5. Standard: You pay $265 before the plan begins to pay.
6. In 2007 and beyond, these amounts will change. For example, the 2006 deductible amount of $250 will be $265 in 2007. The current coverage limit is $2,250 in 2006, in 2007 it will be $2,400. The out-of-pocket threshold in 2006 has been $3,600, it will be $3,850 in 2007. The total covered drug spending requirement in 2006 is $5,100, it will be $5,451.25 in 2007.

Coverage

There may be a tiered co-payment in place. In this case, there will be a set amount you pay for drugs; it is different for each tier (level). As an example, you may pay co-payments that are lower for generic drugs, and higher amounts for brand name drugs.

Type of Additional Coverage Offered in Drug Coverage Gap (the "Donut Hole")

All plans offer coverage until you hit a limit of $2,400 in total drug costs and all plans offer coverage when your out-of-pocket costs exceed $3,850. Some plans *offer* coverage during the gap between $2,400 in total costs and $3,850 in out-of-pocket costs. Plans may pay for differing drugs in the "donut hole" gap:

- Generics Only—Plan covers generic drugs in coverage gap
- Generics and Brands—Plan may cover both generic and brand drugs in coverage gap

Most Commonly Used Drugs

Out of the number of Top 100 Drugs on Formulary, how many of the most commonly used 100 drugs does the plan cover? These are the most commonly used drugs in seniors on average. Ask your pharmacist to help you with the answer to this question. The Medicare website will also have some information to help you: www.medicare.gov.

Convenience

Will it be easy for you to obtain your prescription medications? Might you have the choice of a mail service option? That is, will you be able to get your drugs in the mail and possibly save money and time? You may also be able to obtain a larger quantity on your prescriptions if you are required to use a mail order pharmacy.

Network Pharmacy

Each Part D drug plan has a network of pharmacies for members to use to fill prescriptions. This network may be national in scope and include many pharmacies across the state where you live or across the nation. Others may have a much smaller network of eligible pharmacies for you to use. This is information that is available from each plan. The best way to find the answer to the question of which pharmacies can be used, is to ask your pharmacist where you obtain your current prescriptions. They will easily be able to advise you as to whether you have many pharmacies to choose from or a much smaller number of potential pharmacies in which to obtain your medications.

Medicare Advantage Plans (This Material Is Adapted from the www.cms.gov Website)

The second type of prescription plan that will be available to you is what is termed a Medicare Advantage plan. There are several things that you can decide about the Medicare Advantage Plans and the differences between them. Each plan will provide an overview of important information, how much the premiums are monthly, and what the Medicare Advantage plan will pay for and what it covers. Of the two basic types of plans, the Medicare Advantage plans have by far been the more confusing of the options. In some cases people eligible for extra help or those with both Medicare and Medicaid benefits have been assigned to a plan automatically. People simply do not understand what these managed care options mean for their care. Also, in many parts of the Midwest and Far West do not have options available to them for Medicare Advantage coverage. On the Medicare website and in their written materials, there will numerous things that you can consider.

There are two basic types of plans providing prescription coverage under Medicare Part D, they are prescription drug plans (PDPs) and Medicare Advantage plans.

Location by County

There will be a listing of the counties in a state where a plan is available.

Organization Name

The name of the company offering the Medicare drug plan. Some organizations may offer more than one Medicare drug plan.

Plan Name: The Name of the Medicare Dug Plan

This will be the name of the company offering the Medicare drug plan. Some sponsoring organizations may offer more than one Medicare drug plan. It must be noted that these differing plans will have different coverage options as well.

How Will This Program Work and How Can I Determine What Is Best for Me?

15

Type of Medicare Advantage Plan

- HMO (health maintenance organization): A type of health plan in which you generally must see doctors and hospitals on the plan's list (network) except in an emergency. You also need a referral to see a specialist.
- Local PPO (preferred provider organization): A type of health plan in which you pay less if you use doctors and hospitals on the plan's list (network). You can go to any doctor or hospital not on the plan's list, but it will usually cost more. You do not need a referral to see a specialist.
- Regional PPO (preferred provider organization): A type of health plan in which you pay less if you use doctors and hospitals on the plan's list (network). You can go to any doctor or hospital not on the plan's list, but it will usually cost more. You do not need a referral to see a specialist. A regional PPO has a larger service area than a local PPO.
- Private Fee-for-Service (FFS): A type of health plan in which you can go to any doctor or hospital that accepts the terms of the plan's payment. You do not need a referral to see a specialist.
- Medicare Cost Plan: A type of health plan in which you can use doctors and hospitals on the plan's list (network). However, unlike Medicare Advantage Plans, if you get services from a non-network provider, they are covered under the Original Medicare Plan. Coverage in Medicare Cost Plans can include prescription drug coverage. These plans do not provide free additional benefits or savings on your Medicare Part B or prescription drug coverage premiums. There are a limited number of Medicare Cost Plans.
- Demonstration Plan (Demo Plan): These plans are special projects that test possible future improvements in Medicare coverage, costs, and quality of care. They may include several or many types of services that are not currently available for the majority of Medicare recipients.

Cost

- Beneficiary Total Premium: The total amount you would pay the plan each month for your health care and prescription drug coverage. You do not pay an additional amount for drug coverage with these plans; it is all included in your premium paid monthly.
- Beneficiary Drug Premium: The amount of the beneficiary total premium that goes toward the drug coverage portion of the Medicare Advantage plan. This is not an additional amount you pay.
  - Important: Please note, if you notice a dash in the "Beneficiary Drug Premium" column under descriptors of these plans, this means that these plans do not offer prescription drug coverage.
- Drug Deductible: The amount you pay before the drug plan begins to pay.
- Zero: You do not have to pay anything before the plan begins to pay.
- Reduced: You pay less than $265 before the plan begins to pay.
- Standard: You pay $265 before the plan begins to pay.

Coverage

- Includes Tiered Co-payments for Drugs: The set amount you pay for drugs is different for each tier (level). This tiering was discussed in Chapter 1, and is displayed in Table 1–2.
- Type of Additional Coverage Offered in Drug Coverage Gap: All plans offer coverage until you hit a limit of $2,400 in total drug costs and all plans offer coverage when your out-of-pocket costs exceed $3,850. Some plans offer coverage during the gap between $2,400 in total costs and $3,850 in out-of-pocket costs.
  - Generics Only: Plan covers generic drugs in coverage gap (donut hole).
  - Generics and Brands: Plan covers generic and brand drugs in coverage gap (donut hole).

How Will This Program Work and How Can I Determine What Is Best for Me?

Number of Top 100 Drugs on Formulary

As noted previously, how many of the most commonly used 100 drugs does the plan cover? This is important and I encourage you to determine if your current drugs are covered within a specific plan. Ask your pharmacist to help you with the answer to this question. The Medicare website will also have some information to help you: www.medicare.gov.

Convenience

Gettng your drugs in the mail (mail order) will be an attractive option for some. This is not a program that will appeal to others, especially if you cannot use your normal pharmacy and are forced to use mail order pharmacies.

Network Pharmacy

Just like with the Prescription Drug Plans (PDPs), each Medicare Advantage Part D drug plan has a network of pharmacies for members to use to fill prescriptions. This network may be national in scope and include many pharmacies across the state where you live or across the nation. Others may have a much smaller network of eligible pharmacies for you to use. This is information that is available from each plan. The best way to find the answer to the question of which pharmacies can be used, is to ask your pharmacist where you obtain your current prescriptions. They will easily be able to advise you as to whether you have many pharmacies to choose from or a much smaller number of potential pharmacies in which to obtain your medications.

General Issues Across Both Prescription Drug Plans and Medicare Advantage Plans

Maintaining Drug Coverage for Major Diseases

One aspect of the Medicare Part D Program that Medicare officials have put in place is ensuring that certain drugs are covered. This has been in place whether you have a prescription drug plan or a Medicare Advantage plan. This is only fair and is a very nice component of this new plan. Basically, Medicare officials did not want anyone to be slighted in this new plan. In order to protect against discrimination, CMS has reviewed six drug classes (types of drugs to treat the same condition) and made the stipulation that certain drugs will be covered. These drug classes include the following types of drugs:

- Antidepressants
  - Drug to treat depression
- Antipsychotics
  - Drugs to treat certain mental disorders
- Anticonvulsants
  - Drugs to control seizures
- Antiretrovirals
  - Drugs for autoimmune deficiency syndrome (AIDS). These are drugs for HIV positive patients
- Antineoplastics
  - Drugs to treat cancer of one type or another
- Immunosuppressants
  - Drugs that are prescribed when a patient has had an organ transplant. These drugs work to stop the problem of organ rejection.

The best way to find the answer to the question of which pharmacies can be used, is to ask your pharmacist where you obtain your current prescriptions. They will easily be able to advise you as to whether you have many pharmacies to choose from or a much smaller number of potential pharmacies in which to obtain your medications.

Extra Help for Those with Extra Needs

Because of your financial situation, you may qualify for extra help with your prescription needs. For example, if you currently receive medicines through the Medicaid program in your state, you will automatically be enrolled in a Medicare Part D Plan. Instead of receiving your drug coverage from your Medicaid insurance, you will now receive your medicines through Medicare Part D insurance. There has been confusion about this part of Medicare Part D, so if you are reading this and do not quite understand it, you are not alone! There will be sections in this book in the next chapters that will help you decide if you are eligible for extra help with your medicine needs. Also, please see Appendix A: General summary of the issues related to Medicare Part D and Chapter 3 for ways to determine if you meet the criterion for extra help.

The technical term used by Medicare for this special help is termed a low-income subsidy (LIS). CMS estimates that there are 13.2 million seniors that are eligible for this help, so be sure you can do what you need to do to determine if you, too, qualify!

What Do I Do Now?

Learning About Different Plans

You will need to spend time examining what options are available to you in your region of the country. There will be several options available to you. I encourage you to have someone help you at this point. You will need to know the exact spelling of the drugs that you take. If you take a drug that has an extended release form that you take once a day, know what this is. So, those "XL," "SR," and "CR" letters that follow the name of your drug are very important for you to know. Some plans might cover some of the forms of the drug that you take, but may not cover the exact formulation that you take. Keep looking until you can determine if the plan you choose will cover your present drugs. For some prescriptions, there are abbreviated spellings of the drug on the prescription container that you receive. Find out the completed spelling for of the drugs you take.

Know When You Need to Sign Up for Coverage

Find out the completed spelling of all of the drugs you take. Have your pharmacist help you with this – you will need this when you look your drugs up on a plan formulary.

Be sure to know the times of the year you are eligible to sign up for coverage. Also, be aware that the plans available in 2007 for your consideration will be available to consider in October 2006.

You also have certain rights as a Medicare Insurance participant. These rights are to protect you should something happen to you in the program or to you as a patient that you do not feel right about. Please see Figure 2–1 for a description of what these rights are and what you need to do if you require some assistance with your rights. Figure 2-1 is from the Medicare website and describes what your rights are in the Medicare Part D Program. This copy of Description of Your Rights Under Medicare Part D Drug Coverage explains what you can expect from providers (pharmacists and physicians), and what to do if you have been told that your prescriptions are not covered under your Medicare Part D Plan. You contact the prescription drug plan to explain why your particular drugs have not been included in your benefit. These rights include your ability to obtain written information if you request it. If you are a told that a particular drug you take is not covered under Medicare Part D, you have a right to petition to have the drug added. You also have the right to have the response of the prescription drug plan in writing explaining the situation and decision to you. If you or your doctor feel that you should be on a certain drug, and have very good reasons for suggesting this, do not take no for an answer. Keep trying and proceed through the process to obtain the answer to your question. You owe this to yourself to obtain the information you need and the proper therapy that you need.

Medicare Prescription Drug Coverage and Your Rights

You have the right to get a written explanation from your Medicare drug plan if:

- Your doctor or pharmacist tells you that your Medicare drug plan will not cover a prescription drug in the amount or form prescribed by your doctor.
- You are asked to pay a different cost-sharing amount than you think you are required to pay for a prescription drug.

The Medicare drug plan's written explanation will give you the specific reasons why the prescription drug is not covered and will explain how to request an appeal if you disagree with the drug plan's decision.

You **also have the right to ask** your Medicare drug plan **for an exception** if:

- You believe you need a drug that is not on your drug plan's list of covered drugs. The list of covered drugs is called a "formulary;" or

- You believe you should get a drug you need at a lower cost-sharing amount.

What you need to do:
- Contact your Medicare drug plan to ask for a written explanation about why a prescription is not covered or to ask for an exception if you believe you need a drug that is not on your drug plan's formulary or believe you should get a drug you need at a lower cost-sharing amount.
- Refer to the benefits booklet you received from your Medicare drug plan or call 1-800-MEDICARE to find out how to contact your drug plan.
- When you contact your Medicare drug plan, be ready to tell them:

   1. The prescription drug(s) that you believe you need.
   2. The name of the pharmacy or physician who told you that the prescription drug(s) is not covered.
   3. The date you were told that the prescription drug(s) is not covered.

According to the Paperwork Reduction Act of 1995, no persons are required to respond to a collection of information unless it displays a valid OMB control number. The valid OMB control number for this information collection is 0938-0975. The time required to distribute this information collection once it has been completed is one minute per response, including the time to select the preprinted form, and hand it to the enrollee. If you have any comments concerning the accuracy of the time estimates or suggestions for improving this form, please write to CMS, 7500 Security Boulevard, Attn: PRA Reports Clearance Officer, Baltimore, Maryland 21244-1850.
No. CMS-10147

Figure 2–1   Description of Your Rights Under Medicare Part D Drug Coverage
Approved OMB #0938-0975
Source: www.cms.gov

CHAPTER 3

Are You Eligible for Extra Help with the Medicare Part D Program?

Extra Help Is Available for Many

You Will Need to Do Several Things to Make Sure You Get the Help You Deserve

There is extra help available for many seniors to help pay premiums and costs of the medications in Medicare Part D. The key here is to know where to find the information you need. It is also important that you realize that you can ask for help and receive information. Sources of help may include:

- Family
- Friends
- State resources where you live
- Medicaid offices
- Social Security Administration offices

Please do not be embarrassed if you have to ask someone to help you with figuring out just what to do with Medicare Part D.

If you do qualify for extra assistance, Medicare may help you further by:

- Reducing the initial deductible you have to pay (prescription drug costs) to no more than $50 (Medicare Part has a standard deductible of $265)
- You may not have to pay a monthly premium for the Medicare Part D insurance, or your amount to pay may be less than the usual $32 or so per month
- Limiting co-payments (per prescription) to 15 percent
- You may not have a gap in your coverage for prescriptions. You will not have a "donut hole" where you have to pay for drugs before your coverage resumes.

In practical terms, this extra help will save you a lot of money. Your initial monthly premium may be reduced. Then you will have to pay $50 for drugs before Medicare Part begins to pay for your medications. Until you reach the catastrophic coverage limit, you will pay 15% of the cost of your medications. Medicare will pay for the remaining 85%. When you then qualify for catastrophic coverage, you will pay about $2.00 for each generic prescription, and $5.00 for each brand name prescription (these are drugs for which there is not a generic available) you need to take. For more information about this, please check with your pharmacists or the prescription plan.

This is a government program, so you will have to provide information to verify your eligibility. When you apply for extra assistance, you will need to fill out forms that ask what your income is. You will also need to list what financial resources you have. Finally, you will be asked to sign the form indicating that your answers are true. The Social Security Administration will then verify your answers by examining records from the Internal Revenue Service. Please do not let this paperwork discourage you. You can visit the Social Security Administration (SSA) website (www.ssa.gov/prescriptionhelp) for more information. You can also seek help at your local Social Security Office. You can also call the Social

Security Administration (SSA) toll-free at 1-800-772-1213 and ask for an application or for help with the forms.

If you apply, are successful, and receive extra benefits, you can sign up for Medicare Part D anytime of the year. You will *not* be assessed a penalty on premiums paid per month.

Where can you apply? There are several places where you can seek the extra help coverage:

- At your local Social Security office (the SSA will also take an application over phone)
- Through your state Medicaid office
- Through programs called state health insurance assistance programs (SHIPs)
- Through the SSA website (www.ssa.gov/prescription-help).

This is a government program, so you will have to provide information to verify your eligibility. When you apply for extra assistance, you will need to fill out forms that ask what your income is. You will also need to list what financial resources you have. Finally, you will be asked to sign the form indicating that your answers are true.

The Social Security Administration Will Mail Applications to Many Eligible People

The Social Security Administration routinely mails applications to potentially eligible individuals. As noted, you can also find the forms and additional information on the SSA Web site at www.socialsecurity.gov, or simply call the SSA (1-800-772-1213) to request the form. You will have to be patient when you call this number. There is an automated answering system, and you will have to enter several things or say several things. The initial message will be to contact CMS or www.medicare.gov. Continue through the system, but please do not get frustrated and hang up. You will be finally asked to say: "Medicare Part D," you can then receive the information that you need from the Social Security Administration.

Once a beneficiary qualifies for this extra help, he or she needs to enroll in a Medicare low income-subsidy prescription drug plan. But again, you will not be charged a penalty if your time to sign up has passed. You will not be charged extra if you qualify for extra help.

If you apply, are successful, and receive extra benefits, you can sign up for Medicare Part D anytime of the year. You will not be assessed a penalty on premiums paid per month!

Extra Help in Addition to Regular Assistance

There is an option for some prescription drug plans to offer a supplemental policy in addition to the regular basic policy. In this instance, the premium supplement may pay for drugs not normally covered in Medicare Part D. Drugs such as benzodiazepines are not required to be covered in any Part D plan. Benzodiazepines are drugs such as Valium® (diazepam), Xanax ® (alprazolam), or Halcion® (triazolam) for example. A supplemental premium will add an additional cost to the amount you pay each month. Here is how it works. Say you live in a state and the low-income premium subsidy amount is $25.00. The prescription drug plan has a basic premium of $20.00 per month. The supplemental premium amount is $10.00. Medicare will pay the $20.00 basic premium because it is less than the regional amount ($25.00). A person who obtains the extra help and chooses to sign up for the premium policy as well will pay the $10.00 supplemental premium with their own funds. Another example would be a case where the regional subsidy is $25.00 and the basic plan premium is $30.00 per month. The premium policy amount is $10.00. Medicare will pay the $25.00 subsidy, leaving the person to pay $15.00 per month for the additional coverage ($30.00 - $25.00 paid by Medicare + $10.00 supplemental premium cost = $15.00 per month).

What if I cannot afford a prescription drug plan and in the past I received Medicaid assistance with my medication costs?

How Do I Find Out if I Qualify?

You may qualify if you have limited income and resources. Limited income in August as of 2006 (this may change in the future as adjustments are made) is $14,700 for a single individual and $19,800 for a married couple. If your income is higher, you may still qualify for extra help. For example, if you support family members who live with you or you have some earnings from a job. Also, if you live in Alaska or Hawaii these limits are different, so you may qualify if your income is higher.

You may also receive help from other sources. These additional means of support do not count as part of your income! They should not be entered in the total for your income estimate. These other sources include:

- Food stamp assistance
- Home energy assistance
- Housing assistance
- Disaster assistance (help during Hurricane Katrina for example)
- Earned income tax credits
- Victim compensation
- Scholarships and/or educational grants.

When you are filling out the required forms, limited resources refers to below $10,000 for an individual or less than $20,000 for a married couple. You can also add an extra $1,500 per person if you will use funds for burial purposes.

Please note that the following do not count as resources:

- Your primary residence
- Your personal possessions
- Your vehicles
- Things like jewelry or home furnishings—things you could not easily convert to cash
- Rental property that you need for self-support. This might include land that you use to grow produce for home consumption.
- Non-business property essential for your self-sufficiency
- Up to $1,500 for singles, $3,000 for couples living together or cash life insurance policies
- Burial plots

Persons with Medicaid Coverage

People with limited income and resources will qualify for extra help paying their premium and for some of the cost of their prescriptions. If you are on Medicare and receiving full Medicaid benefits (including prescription drug coverage) you are automatically enrolled to get extra help in a prescription drug plan. This replacement coverage began January 1, 2006. The following Table 3–1 explains what you will pay with the basic Medicare prescription drug plan.

What If You Previously Were on Medicaid and Medicaid Paid for Your Medications?

You may be receiving Supplemental Security Income Benefits. This supplement is a monthly amount paid by the Social Security Administration to persons with a limited income and resources who are blind, disabled, or age 65 years or older. Please note that this is not the typical Social Security payment you receive monthly. You will be placed in a Medicare Part D Plan automatically. Your coverage will begin the first day that your Medicare Part A and Part B are in effect. You will be enrolled in a plan that pays your medication costs effective the very first day. You will also be able to switch plans at any point should you wish to.

Table 3–1 Individuals on Medicare with Medicaid Prescription Benefits		
	Living in a nursing home or medical institution	Income below $9,570 for an individual; $12,830 for a couple
Premium	$0	$0
Deductible	$0	$0
Co-payment	$0	$1 for each generic prescription, $3 for each brand name prescription
Catastrophic Coverage	$0	You pay nothing after your total drug expenses reach $5,100

Do You Have a Limited Income but Do Not Qualify for Medicaid Coverage for Your Prescription Drugs?

You may have both Medicare and Medicaid coverage, but you do not have Medicaid coverage for your prescription needs. Please see Table 3–2. You may still qualify for extra help with your prescriptions if your income is below $14,355 if you are single and $19,245 if you are married and your assets are below $11,500 for singles and $23,000 for married couples. The table below explains the benefits and how you qualify.

If you think you qualify for extra help with drug plan costs, you must follow a two-step process:

1. First, you must *apply for the extra help* paying prescription plan costs; contact your local Social Security office. Enrollment can be done by mail, by telephone, or online.
2. Then, you must *enroll in* a *Medicare prescription drug plan* that meets your needs.

Pharmaceutical Assistance Programs

In recent years, many pharmaceutical companies have either by themselves or together provided assistance programs to

Table 3–2	People with Medicare and Medicaid without Drug Coverage	
Income	Income below** $12,920/individual $17,321/couple	Income below $14,355/individual* $19,245/couple*
Assets	Below $6,000/individual $9,000/couple	Below $11,500/individual $23,000/couple
Premium	$0	premium based upon income
Deductible	$0	$50
Co-payment	$2 for generic prescriptions, $5 for brand name prescription	15% coinsurance
	You pay nothing after your total drug expenses reach $5,000	$2 for generic prescription, $5 for brand name prescription after drug expenses reach $5,100

*2005 Income Requirement; ** Includes individuals enrolled in SSI and Medicare Savings Programs.

help defray the cost of medications they manufacture. Individual states have also in some cases provided assistance to seniors who could not afford the drugs they take. Perhaps you have benefited from these programs. Early in 2006, CMS indicated that these "helping" programs could continue to provide support for individuals. However, the support cannot be part of the Medicare Part D program. The help must be outside of the Medicare benefit. So what does all this mean?

You will need to carefully examine all your drugs. If there are some drugs that can be provided to you by way of these assistance programs, please know which ones can and cannot be obtained through these plans. You will have to contact the company or you can have your doctor or pharmacist help you as well. You then may have other drugs that are not covered by these assistance programs, but that you still need to take. These are the prescriptions that you will submit for coverage under Medicare Part D. This may seem like a lot of work, and it is! But, you can save yourself quite a bit of money by looking into this option. If you are just starting on a new prescription, you might also ask your doctor to provide one from those that qualify for extra help from manufacturers. Please see Appendix B for a listing of pharmaceutical assistance programs sponsored by the pharmaceutical industry.

There are also several states that continue to have assistance programs. I wish all states would! Find out from helping agencies in your state if there is such a program where you live. By all means, take advantage of these programs any way you can. Please see Appendix C for a listing of states with these programs as of August 9, 2006.

You should do everything mentioned in this book to help you choose which plan is best for you. If you need help with the complex information, ask for some assistance from a family member or friend. No one will be able to help you until you ask them for some help and assistance. It is important for you to realize that this is a very complicated program. No one has all the right answers. Certainly, no one can learn what they need to do without some preparation. Please do not be embarrassed if you have to ask someone to help you figure out just what to do with Medicare Part D.

The following pages contain excerpts from the pamphlets and brochures that have been provided by the Social Security Administration or by CMS to help those with extra needs know how and where to turn for extra help. This help will save you money, so please check out these resources and see if you can obtain the most help that you possibly can.

The pamphlets that appeared on the previous and next two pages provide information for individuals to determine if they are eligible for extra assistance. This brochure describes what individuals need to do to assess whether or not they have extra assistance available to them.

This is the Social Security Administration forms to apply for extra assistance. Your local SSA office will have these forms and the staff there can help you fill them out if necessary. The forms on the following pages are also available to you to help you with questions you might have about Medicare Part D.

The brochure on the following pages provides quick tips on the Medicare Part D program for persons with limited incomes. These individuals will be able to receive additional monetary assistance.

Chapter Figures

On the following pages, there are a series of informational brochures that are provided by the United States Social Security Administration. Figure 3–1 is a copy of a poster that has been produced by the Social Security Administration which highlights phone numbers and the website providing further information to seniors with limited incomes. Figure 3–2 provides a step-by-step description of what needs to be done if individuals qualify for extra help. Figure 3–3 provides information on exactly what to include and not include in the application for extra assistance in the Medicare Part D program. Figure 3–4 provides information about what information is necessary when applying for extra help in the program. Also in Figure 3–4, a worksheet is provided for seniors or their helpers to list necessary information when applying for extra help. Figure 3–5 presents information seniors should know about the Medicare Part D program.

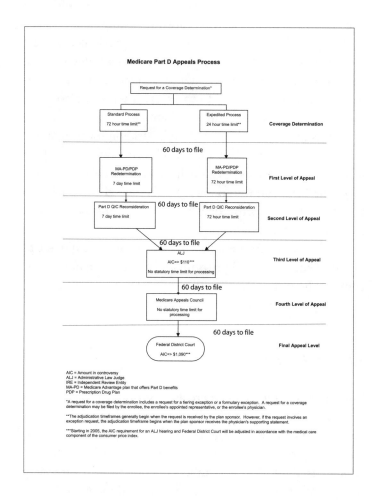

Figure 3-1   Poster Promoting Medicare Part D
Source: Social Security Administration

★ ★ TIP SHEET ★ ★

Information Partners Can Use on:

Next Steps for People with Medicare Who Qualify for Extra Help

New Medicare Prescription Drug Coverage   **As of May 2006**

This tip sheet explains what people with Medicare should do after they receive a letter from the Social Security Administration (SSA) or their state telling them that they qualify for extra help.

Step 1: Learn about Options

To get extra help paying for prescriptions, they will need to choose and join a Medicare drug plan. They have three options to consider.

Option 1: They can join a Medicare drug plan on their own. They can visit www.medicare.gov on the web or call 1-800-MEDICARE (1-800-633-4227) for help comparing plans and joining a plan that works for them. TTY users should call 1-877-486-2048. When comparing these plans, they should find out which plans cover the prescriptions they take and what pharmacies they can use to fill their prescriptions. If they choose and join a drug plan, Medicare won't enroll them in a plan.

Option 2: Medicare will enroll them in a Medicare drug plan. If they don't join a Medicare drug plan or call 1-800-MEDICARE and decline Medicare prescription drug coverage, Medicare will enroll them in a Medicare drug plan and send them a letter telling them when their coverage will begin.

Option 3: They can decline to have Medicare enroll them in a plan. They can choose not to join. If they currently have other drug coverage, it may be as good as or better than Medicare prescription drug coverage. They may want to keep their current coverage and decline enrollment from Medicare. If they don't want Medicare drug coverage, they can call 1-800-MEDICARE (1-800-633-4227) and tell them they don't want to enroll. Remember, if they decline, they won't be enrolled in a Medicare drug plan now.

Step 2: Review Other Current Prescription Drug Coverage

If they have, or are eligible for other types of prescription coverage, they should read all the materials they get from their insurer or plan provider. Examples of other types of prescription drug coverage include coverage from a current or former employer or union, TRICARE, the Department of Veteran's Affairs, or a Medigap (Medicare Supplement Insurance) policy.

continued on back

Figure 3–2   Next Steps for People with Medicare Who Qualify for Extra Help

Source: Social Security Administration

Are You Eligible for Extra Help With Medicare Part D Program?

They should talk to their benefits administrator, insurer, or plan provider. Joining a Medicare drug plan may affect their current prescription drug coverage. It may also affect coverage their spouse or other dependents may be getting if they are covered through that plan. Their current coverage may be as good as or better than Medicare prescription drug coverage. They may not need to join a Medicare drug plan. They may need to decline this enrollment from Medicare by calling 1-800-MEDICARE (1-800-633-4227) to keep their current coverage. TTY users should call 1-877-486-2048.

Step 3: Decide Which Option is Best

They need to consider their three options carefully. If they don't join a plan on their own or call 1-800-MEDICARE (1-800-633-4227) to decline Medicare prescription drug coverage, Medicare will enroll them in a drug plan. They may pay a premium fee to the plan each month. If they get a bill and don't want the plan, they should call the plan or 1-800-MEDICARE to decline the coverage. If they want to keep the plan Medicare enrolls them in, they don't need to do anything. They have Medicare prescription drug coverage to help them save money now and protect their future prescription needs.

Switching Drug Plans

If they join a Medicare drug plan on their own, Medicare will honor their choice and not enroll them in another drug plan. But if they don't join a drug plan on their own and Medicare enrolls them in one, they can still switch plans. They can switch to a different Medicare drug plan at least once until the end of the calendar year, and once each year after, between November 15 and December 31. To join a different Medicare drug plan, they should call the new plan to find out how to join. Joining a different plan will disenroll them from their current plan. Their new plan coverage would start the following month.

Note: In special circumstances, Medicare may give them other opportunities to switch to another Medicare prescription drug plan. For example, if they permanently move out of their drug plan's service area; if the plan stops offering prescription drug coverage; or if they enter, live in, or leave a nursing home.

> **For more information about Medicare prescription drug coverage**
> - Visit www.medicare.gov on the web and select "Search Tools" to get personalized drug plan information.
> - Call 1-800-MEDICARE (1-800-633-4227). TTY users should call 1-877-486-2048.
> - Call your State Health Insurance Assistance Program (SHIP) for free personalized health insurance counseling. See your copy of the "Medicare & You" handbook or call 1-800-MEDICARE for their telephone number.

Figure 3–2   (continued)

★ ★ TIP SHEET ★ ★

Information Partners Can Use on:

Helping People with Medicare Apply for Extra Help

New Medicare Prescription Drug Coverage   **As of March 2006**

You continue to be a valuable resource in helping people with Medicare apply for **extra help** paying their Medicare drug plan costs. A person may qualify for extra help if they have limited **income** and **resources**. Read below for more detailed information.

- **Limited income** (below $14,700 for an individual or $19,800 for a married couple living together). **Even if their annual income is higher, a person still may be able to get some help with their prescription costs.** Some examples where income may be higher include if a person or their spouse

  — support other family members, who live with them, or

  — have earnings from work, or

  — live in Alaska or Hawaii.

The following cash payments **don't count as income:**

- Food stamp assistance
- Home energy assistance
- Medical care assistance
- Housing assistance
- Disaster assistance
- Earned income tax credit payments
- Victim's compensation
- Scholarships and education grants

Continued on back

Figure 3–3   Helping People with Medicare Apply for Extra Help
Source: Social Security Administration

Are You Eligible for Extra Help With Medicare Part D Program?

★

- Limited resources (below $10,000 for an individual or $20,000 for a married couple living together). These resource limits can be slightly higher (an additional $1,500 per person) if a person will use some of the money for burial expenses.

  The following items don't count as a resource:
  - Your primary residence
  - Your personal possessions
  - Your vehicle(s)
  - Resources you could not easily convert to cash, such as jewelry or home furnishings
  - Property you need for self-support, such as rental property or land you use to grow produce for home consumption
  - Non-business property essential to your self-support
  - Up to $1,500 (or $3,000 if you are married and living with your spouse) of the cash value of life insurance policies
  - Burial spaces

Social Security has a simple application process to help people with Medicare apply for extra help. There are several ways for people with Medicare to apply for extra help:

- Apply online at www.socialsecurity.gov.
- Get an application or apply over the phone by calling Social Security at 1-800-772-1213. TTY users should call 1-800-325-0778.
- Attend a community event sponsored by Social Security or a civic or service organization where they can complete an application. Questions about extra help will be answered at these events. Staff from Social Security's 1,300 field offices are out in local communities taking applications at locations such as senior centers, libraries and places of worship.
- Visit a local Social Security field office.

For more information about applying for extra help with your Medicare drug plan costs, call Social Security at 1-800-772-1213 or visit www.socialsecurity.gov/prescriptionhelp on the web.

Figure 3–3   (continued)

What You Need To Complete The Application For Help With Medicare Prescription Drug Plan Costs

2006

Social Security and the Centers for Medicare & Medicaid Services are working together to get you extra help with your prescription drug costs. To determine if you could be eligible for this extra help, Social Security will need to know your income and the value of your savings, investments and real estate (other than your home). You may qualify for extra help if you have:

- Limited income (below $14,700 for an individual or $19,800 for a married couple living together). Even if your annual income is higher, you still may be able to get some help with your monthly premiums, annual deductibles and prescription co-payments. Some examples where your income may be higher include if you or your spouse:

  —Support other family members who live with you;

  —Have earnings from work; or

  —Live in Alaska or Hawaii; and

- Resources limited to $10,000 for an individual or $20,000 for a married couple living together. These resource limits can be slightly higher (an additional $1,500 per person) if you will use some of your money for burial expenses.

What you need to know

Identify the things you own by yourself, with your spouse or with someone else, but **do not** include your home, vehicles, burial plots or personal possessions.

Review all your income.

Gather your records in advance to save time.

Remember that this worksheet is **not** an application. This worksheet can assist you in completing the actual application for extra help.

Documents that will help you prepare in advance include:

- Statements that show your account balances at banks, credit unions or other financial institutions;
- Investment statements;
- Life insurance policy statements;
- Stock certificates;
- Tax returns;
- Pension award letters; and
- Payroll slips.

How you can get more information

If you need an application form, contact Social Security at **1-800-772-1213** (TTY **1-800-325-0778**) and ask for the *Application for Help with Medicare Prescription Drug Plan Costs* (SSA-1020). You can also apply online at *www.socialsecurity.gov*.

To learn more about the Medicare prescription drug plans, call **1-800-MEDICARE** (**1-800-633-4227**) or visit *www.medicare.gov*.

Please continue to the opposite side of the page to complete the worksheet.

(over)

What You Need To Complete The Application For
Help With Medicare Prescription Drug Plan Costs

www.socialsecurity.gov

Are You Eligible for Extra Help With Medicare Part D Program?

Figure 3–4   What You Need to Complete the Application for Help with Medicare Prescription Drug Plan Costs

Source: Social Security Administration

37

We need to know information about your (and your spouse's, if you are married and living together) income and resources:

Name	Social Security Number

Resources	Value
Bank accounts, including checking, savings and certificates of deposit	$ _____
Stocks, bonds, savings bonds, mutual funds, individual retirement accounts (IRAs) or other investments	$ _____
Cash at home or anywhere else	$ _____
Life insurance policies for you (and your spouse, if married and living together)	$ _____

NOTE: *Social Security needs to know how much money you would get **if you cashed in your life insurance policies today**. Check with your insurance company or agent to get the exact cash value. This probably will be less than the amount you are insured for.*

Any real estate other than your home	$ _____

Income	Monthly Amount
Social Security Benefits	$ _____
Railroad Retirement	$ _____
Veterans benefits	$ _____
Other pensions or annuities	$ _____
Alimony	$ _____
Net rental income	$ _____
Workers' compensation	$ _____
Help from other people to pay for household expenses, such as food, mortgage or rent, heating fuel or gas, electricity, water and property taxes	$ _____
Wages	$ _____
Self-employment net earnings	$ _____
Other income	$ _____

You may choose to have someone help you when you do business with Social Security. We will work with that person, just as we would work with you.

www.socialsecurity.gov

Social Security Administration
SSA Publication No. 05-10128
ICN 480068
Unit of Issue - HD (one hundred)
March 2006 (Destroy prior editions)

Figure 3–4   (continued)

What You Should Know About The New Medicare Prescription Drug Plans

How Social Security can help you with the new Medicare prescription drug plans

- Social Security **can help you apply for extra help** paying for your Medicare prescription drug plan costs if you have limited income and resources.
- Social Security **can provide information about the organizations that are available in your community** to help you make choices about enrolling in a plan.
- Social Security **cannot provide advice about or help you choose** which prescription drug plan is best for you.

How you can get help to make a decision on enrolling in a specific prescription drug plan

- You can **call Medicare at 1-800-MEDICARE (1-800-633-4227)**. If you are deaf or hard of hearing, you can call the toll-free **TTY number at 1-877-486-2048.**
- You can visit **www.medicare.gov** on the Internet and use the following tools:
  - □ **Compare Medicare prescription drug plans**—By allowing you to enter personalized information, you can find and compare the prescription drug plans in your state that meet your personal needs and enroll in the prescription drug plan that you select.
  - □ **Formulary Finder**—By allowing you to enter personalized information about the specific medications you take, you can get information to help you find the plans in your state that match your prescription drug needs.

You can contact your State Health Insurance Assistance Program (SHIP)

You can contact one of the following organizations in your area

(over)

What You Should Know About The
New Medicare Prescription Drug Plans

Figure 3–5   What You Should Know About the New Medicare Prescription Drug Plans
Source: Social Security Administration

39

Important information to consider when making a decision to enroll in a specific prescription drug plan

You can **first join a drug plan between November 15, 2005, and May 15, 2006**. In most cases, if you do not join during this period, your next chance to join will be between November 15, 2006, and December 31, 2006, and you may have to pay a penalty. This means you will pay a higher monthly premium for as long as you have Medicare prescription drug coverage.

You do not have to be eligible for the extra help to join a prescription drug plan. The extra help is in addition to the potential savings you may receive if you join a plan.

If you already have prescription drug coverage, you should talk to your plan benefits administrator or insurer before making any changes.

If you already have prescription drug coverage through a Medicare private health plan or other insurance, check with your current plan to see if this coverage is changing.

You should consider these factors when comparing your Medicare drug plan choices

- **Coverage**—Medicare drug plans will cover generic and brand-name drugs. Most plans will have a formulary, which is a list of drugs covered by the plan. This list must always meet Medicare's requirements, but it can change when plans get new information.
- **Cost**—Monthly premiums and your share of the cost of your prescriptions will vary depending on which plan you choose. You also may be eligible for extra help with these costs if you have limited income and resources.

- **Convenience**—Drug plans must contract with pharmacies in your area. Check with the plan to make sure the pharmacies in the plan are convenient to you.
- **Security now and in the future**—Even if you do not take a lot of prescription drugs now, you should consider joining a drug plan in 2006. For most people, joining now means you will pay your lowest possible monthly premium. If you do not join a plan by May 15, 2006, and you do not currently have a drug plan that, on average, covers at least as much as standard Medicare prescription drug coverage, you will have to wait until November 15, 2006, to join. When you do join, you will have to pay a higher monthly premium. You will have to pay a higher monthly premium for as long as you have Medicare prescription drug coverage.

You can join a Medicare prescription drug plan in the following ways

- **By paper application**—Contact the company offering the drug plan you choose and ask for an application. Once you fill out the form, mail or fax it back to the company.
- **On the plan's website**—Visit the drug plan company's website. You may be able to join online.
- **On Medicare's website**—You also will be able to join a drug plan at **www.medicare.gov** on the web using Medicare's online enrollment center.
- **By calling 1-800-MEDICARE**— You can join a drug plan by calling **1-800-MEDICARE (1-800-633-4227)** and talking to a Medicare customer service representative. TTY users should call **1-877-486-2048**.

Social Security Administration
SSA Publication No. 05-10126
ICN 468760
Unit of Issue - HD (one hundred)
November 2005
U.S. GOVERNMENT PRINTING OFFICE: 2005—320–632/00131

Figure 3–5   (continued)

Sources

Helping People with Medicare Apply for Extra Help, Tip Sheet, CMS, 2006.

The Extra Help for the Basic Premium, Tip Sheet, 2006.

www.ssa.gov

http://www.ssa.gov/prescriptionhelp

www.cms.gov

CHAPTER 4

Choosing a Medicare Part D Insurance Drug Plan

Different Plans and Options

Decisions to Sign Up for Medicare Part D

The first thing that you need to consider when looking at Medicare Part D coverage is whether or not you should sign up for coverage. As noted previously, there are several types of coverage available to you (1). There are numerous prescription drug plans available to you, and there may or may not be a Medicare Advantage plan available in your area. There are some rural parts of the country that will not have a Medicare Advantage plan available for Medicare recipients. In this case, you will have the option of prescription drug plans available to you, and only these types of plans. Please see Figure 4–1 for a depiction of the decision process you might use to decide about Medicare Part D.

If you currently have drug coverage, you may not need to sign up for coverage. If your coverage is not as good as the Medicare Part D option, you should sign up for coverage. The term for this is creditable coverage. If you do not sign up for coverage when you are eligible, and decide to later, you will pay an extra amount each month for your delaying in signing up. Look at the diagram below to see what you might

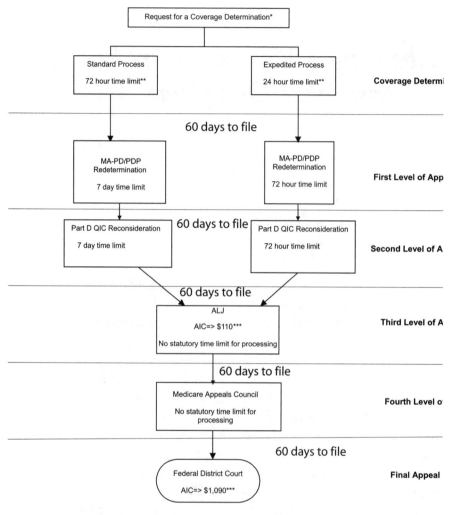

Medicare Part D Appeals Process

Request for a Coverage Determination*

Standard Process
72 hour time limit**

Expedited Process
24 hour time limit**

Coverage Determi

60 days to file

MA-PD/PDP
Redetermination
7 day time limit

MA-PD/PDP
Redetermination
72 hour time limit

First Level of App

Part D QIC Reconsideration
7 day time limit

60 days to file

Part D QIC Reconsideration
72 hour time limit

Second Level of A

60 days to file

ALJ
AIC=> $110***
No statutory time limit for processing

Third Level of A

60 days to file

Medicare Appeals Council
No statutory time limit for
processing

Fourth Level o

60 days to file

Federal District Court
AIC=> $1,090***

Final Appeal

AIC = Amount in controversy
ALJ = Administrative Law Judge
IRE = Independent Review Entity
MA-PD = Medicare Advantage plan that offers Part D benefits
PDP = Prescription Drug Plan

*A request for a coverage determination includes a request for a tiering exception or a formulary exception. A request for a coverage determination may be filed by the enrollee, the enrollee's appointed representative, or the enrollee's physician.

**T

Figure 4–1   Decision Process About Medicare Part D

need to do when considering your options for Medicare Part D drug coverage. If you currently receive Medicaid coverage for your drugs, you will be enrolled automatically in a prescription drug plan that will now pay for your prescription drugs. If you have benefits from the Veterans' Administration (VA) for medication needs, you will continue to receive your medications from the VA. If you do not have coverage for your prescription drugs from other sources, then you are eligible to sign up for Medicare Part D. This is when you look at the plans available to you in your state where you live. The plans will differ in what drugs they cover. Here, it is important to make sure you can obtain your drugs that you need and want to take. This will take a close look at many things. It may be that you pay a little more of a premium each month for coverage, but you might have more drugs covered for less money. Other plans may have a low premium in comparison, but may not cover the drugs that you need at price that is competitive.

Low premiums do not necessarily mean that you will pay less for your drugs, it may be just the opposite!

When making your decisions about Medicare Part D, the first one to make is whether to sign up for the program or not. After you make the decision to sign up, there are other things that you have to decide. There are the plans and what it is they can offer you, and for what price. There are two basic categories of Medicare Part D prescription options. One is termed a prescription drug plan and the second is called a Medicare Advantage plan. These are two very different options. Let's explore what they are and what the differences are. Basically, you need to make the decision that is the best one for you and for your health needs.

The Medicare Prescription Drug Plans

The prescription drug plans are what are termed "stand alone" plans. These plans provide prescription drug coverage if you sign up for it. This coverage is in addition to the services you obtain from Medicare Part A and Medicare Part B.

The plans will differ in what drugs they cover. Here it is important to make sure you can obtain your drugs that you need and want to take.

The two types of Medicare Part D Plans are prescription drug plans or Medicare Advantage plans.

Choosing a Medicare Part D Insurance Drug Plan

45

There are many different prescription drug plans that are offered in the Medicare Part D program. Each of these plans has to meet the basic requirements set forth by the Medicare program for these plans. The numbers of plans available to you vary from state to state. One program in one state may be different from plans available to you in other regions of the United States. These plans provide prescription drug coverage that adds to the traditional Medicare coverage for hospital and outpatient medical care. You will, on average, have around 40 plans from which to choose the one right for you. You might also currently be enrolled in other Medicare health insurance plans, such as:

- Medicare private fee-for-service plans
- Medicare cost plans
- Medicare savings acount plans

You will need to make sure if you have these last 3 types of plans whether the prescription drug plans will be able to provide drug coverage for you if you sign up. Check with the current plans that provide medical insurance for you in the Medicare program to see if Medicare Part D prescription drug plan you are considering will help with your drug costs.

Medicare Advantage Plans

Medicare advantage plans provide a type of coverage that provides for all your Medicare health care needs under one plan. This coverage includes prescription drug coverage as part of the care provided. These health maintenance organizations (HMOs) or preferred provider organizations (PPOs) offer comprehensive coverage that will include prescription drug coverage. You pay a premium each month for all of these services. There are select physicians, hospitals, and pharmacies that you obtain your health care services from. This is a basic difference between HMOs, PPOs, and traditional fee-for-service care. In fee-for-service plans, you can obtain medical, hospital, and pharmacy care from any number of providers in your area. You are not limited to a select panel of providers from which to obtain your healthcare needs. HMOs and PPOs may also limit which hospitals you can use.

New Members in Drug Plans and What They Can Expect with Their Drug Coverage

Some new members may be taking a drug that is not on the formulary for coverage in the prescription drug plan. In this case, Medicare requires plans to provide a standard 30-day supply of all Medicare-covered drugs for new plan members (transition supply). If you are in a nursing home, the plan must approve a six month (180 day) transition supply. This is required by Medicare even if the prescription is for a drug not the plan formulary. If the drug is on the plan, but is only to be taken after a step therapy is tried, this requirement is waived too. The only exception to this is when a drug is simply not approved for payment by Medicare.

This is a fair process and allows you and your doctor to find another drug to use without forcing this on you. There may be drugs that can work as well, and this extra time will be helpful for both you and your doctor. If there is not such a drug, you and/or your doctor can file an appeal to have the drug covered.

At the beginning of 2007, if you stay on the same plan as in 2006, you will not be able to have a transition supply like you did the year before.

Starting your coverage, but you do not have your prescription drug plan card. In this case, you may need to have prescriptions filled before you obtain your card indicating that you have coverage. What will happen more likely is that your plan information is not available for your pharmacy to access through the computer. So that you will not have to pay for these drugs without being reimbursed you can do several things at the pharmacy.

Choosing a Medicare Part D Insurance Drug Plan

So that you do not have to pay out of pocket for these drugs, what you can do is:

- Take your prescription drug plan confirmation or acknowledgement letter to the pharmacy.
- If you do not have the letter yet, let the pharmacist know what plan you have signed up for. I would suggest that you write the following down before you reach the pharmacy:
  - Your enrollment and confirmation number from the plan
  - Your copy of the enrollment application
  - Your welcome letter from the prescription drug plan

This should allow you to obtain your medications.

Creditable Coverage

This is coverage that you currently have from other plans that is as good or better than the Medicare plans that are available to you. If you have such a plan that is provided to you by an employer, or former employer, and it is a good plan, you should not sign up for the Medicare Part D program. If you sign up for coverage under Medicare Part D, you will be assessed a penalty each month plus the normal monthly premium.

What has happened so far with enrollment trends? CMS has noted the following facts with prescription drug plan enrollment to date:

- Lower premiums are associated with higher enrollment
- Having no deductible is associated with higher enrollment
- Having more drugs on a plans formulary is associated with higher enrollment
- A lower percentage of drugs requiring prior authorization or step therapy is associated with higher enrollment

These relationships are consistent between both PDPs and MA-PDs.

There Are Consequences If You Do Not Sign Up When You Are Eligible

Penalty fees. What if you did not enroll in a Medicare prescription drug plan by May 15, 2006, which is the end of your Initial Enrollment Period (IEP)? You do not have creditable coverage and you wait to enroll in a prescription Part D drug plan in November 2006, during the Annual Coordinated Election Period. The penalty will be 6% because you had six months without creditable coverage, starting with the first month the person would have been covered if he or she had joined a plan by May 15. Therefore, you will have to count the months of June, July, August, September, October, and November.

Since the base national premium in 2007 is $27.35 per month, then your penalty would be $27.35 \times .06 = \$1.64$ per month. This will be added to the premium payment amount. It is calculated by multiplying 1% of the base beneficiary premium by the number of months the person was eligible but not enrolled in a plan, and did not have creditable drug coverage.

The penalty calculation is not based on the premium of the plan the individual is enrolled in. The base beneficiary premium is a national number and can change each year.

Initial Enrollment Periods

An enrollment period gives people one opportunity to join, switch, or drop plans. This applies to the Initial Enrollment Period, Special Enrollment Periods, the Annual Coordinated Election Period, and the Medicare Advantage Open Enrollment Period. Once the change has taken effect, that enrollment period is over for that person. If someone quits a plan, that uses the one opportunity to change for that enrollment period. It is important to remember that enrolling in a new drug plan will automatically disenroll people from their current Medicare plan. This includes individuals who are enrolled in most Medicare Advantage Plans. People do not need to request disenrollment from the current plan unless they want to drop Medicare drug coverage completely. In that case, the individual must request disenrollment by contacting the current plan or 1-800-MEDICARE (1-800-633-4227); TTY users should call 1-877-486-2048. On May 15, 2006, the first Initial Enrollment Period ended for people entitled to Medicare in January 2006 or earlier.

What Happens When People First Become Eligible to Enroll in a Medicare Drug Plan?

All people who become entitled to Medicare after January 2006 have a 7-month Initial Enrollment Period (IEP) for enrollment in Part D:

- They can apply three months before their month of Medicare eligibility. Coverage will begin on the date they become eligible.
- They can apply in their month of eligibility, in which case their Part D coverage will begin on the first of the following month.
- Or they can also apply during the three months after their month of eligibility, with coverage beginning the first of the month after the month they apply.

Some groups of people who become entitled to Medicare will be enrolled in a Part D plan by CMS unless they join a plan on their own.

What Happens If I Go into a Nursing Home?

When you enter a nursing home, either a skilled nursing facility (SNF) or an intermediate care facility (ICF), you have several circumstances with Medicare Part D. You have special enrollment period priveliges. You have packaging that is available through institutional pharmacy providers. More on this is presented in Chapter Eight. If you have dual eligibility with both Medicare and Medicaid, you will not have to pay any cost sharing on your medications. Finally, if you are in a nursing home, you will have a broader formulary for drugs available to you. This means you will have more choices for drugs. The only Medicare recipients eligble for this extra series of items are those who live in either a skilled nursing home or a intermediate care facility. If you live in an assisted living home, you do not have these extra options available to you. It is unfortunate that this qualifier is in place. Some of these addition options for nursing home patients, if available to all, could keep some out of nursing homes.

Refunds for Overcharges

There are situations when you will need to get paid back for Medicare drug plan co-payments, deductibles, and/or premium amounts. This is the case when you fill a prescription that should be covered by the plan before receiving a plan membership card or confirmation letter. In these situations should follow these steps:

- Save your original receipt from the pharmacy after you pay for the prescription
- Call the customer service number on your prescription drug plan membership card, or look on the computer website to find out about you can be paid in this process
- Your plan may have a specific claim submission or reimbursement form that you will need to complete and send in
- Finally, fill out the form and submit it to the plan with the original receipt

Under some circumstances, the pharmacy may be able to resubmit the claim electronically and pay you without going through this process. It is important to know that each time a pharmacy submits a claim electronically, the pharmacy is charged a billing fee.

If *you qualify for the extra help* and you are not charged the correct deductible or co-payment amount, you should follow the same steps above to submit a claim for payment from the plan. If you have dual coverage with both Medicare and Medicaid and you live in a nursing home, you may not have to pay for their prescription drugs. If you are charged co-payments, the long-term care pharmacy providing service to you will work with the plan to resolve the amount of any uncollected co-payments for people who were mistakenly identified as having to pay co-payment amounts. This process will vary between plans, but let the pharmacy involved figure this out for you.

How Can I Pay for My Premiums:

You can pay for your premiums several ways, they include:

- You can mail monthly premium payments to the plan you sign up with
- You can automatically transfer the premium to your plan from your bank accounts, either checking or savings
- You can also have monthly premiums taken out of your monthly Social Security benefit

As is the case with many types of withdrawals, it will take time (a couple of months, depending on what time of the month you sign up) before the Social Security deduction is in effect. The way this works is that two months of your premiums are taken out with the first payment made. Single payments will be deducted thereafter. If you enroll in December of the year, you will probably be billed in February for both the January and February premiums. This is a government program and it may take three or more months for this to be in place! If it is more than three months, you will be contacted to see how you want your premiums deducted.

Medicare Errors in Billing

There have also been glitches in the system! On August, 23, 2006 in an article in the *Wichita Eagle*(2), Kevin Freking reported that over 200,000 Medicare recipients received checks that incorrectly reimbursed them for monthly premiums they have paid for prescription drug coverage in 2006. This confusing situation allows checks of around $215 to be paid to recipients. The checks, which are sure to leave many beneficiaries confused, average about $215. These checks are accompanied by a letter indicating that premiums can no longer be deducted from Social Security checks. Medicare sent out around $50 million in incorrect checks. So, another letter was sent telling people not to cash the checks and that this would not affect their Medicare Part D coverage. The checks were required to be returned by the recipients! Also, correct deductions did not begin again until after October 2006. Unfortunately, several payments were deducted at once leaving many in a lurch.

Maintaining Coverage for Your Drugs

The Medicare program has indicated to prescription drug plans that no plan members will be subject to a discontinuation or reduction in coverage of the drugs they are currently using. This can change if a new generic is available for your prescription. Also, if the United States Food and Drug Administration takes action to have a drug removed from the market, this can change as well. This has been the case for 2006 and will be in place in years 2007 and beyond (4).

Challenging a Prescription Drug Plan Action

Medicare Part D Plans will use several processes to manage their formularies. These include:

- *Multiple drug tiers*—these tiers are different cost levels for different types of drugs (e.g., brand-name drugs, preferred generic, generic)

- *Prior authorization*—Here your doctor contacts the prescription drug plan before your prescription is covered
- *Step therapy*—Here you must try one drug, usually lower in cost, before another, more expensive drug can be used
- *Quantity limits*—The prescription drug plan limit the quantity of drugs you can obtain over a certain period of time

Every prescription drug plan must provide a coverage determination and appeals process to allow you to obtain the prescriptions that are medically necessary to your health.

Appealing Plan Decisions That Are Not in Your Favor

You can appeal a decision by a prescription drug plan that is not in your favor (3). You can appoint a representative, such as your doctor or someone in your family, to request a decision about a drug or to appeal a decision that is not in your favor. Your plan will indicate your options and how you file such appointment information or a letter. If you have someone help with your matters through a power of attorney, they too can request such appeal.

Your doctor can also request expedited or standard coverage determinations or expedited re-determinations. In other cases and for other requests, your doctor will need to be your appointed representative. You and others can be assisted by others to complete forms, gathering evidence, letter writing, and other forms of help. You can request a coverage determination either orally or in writing. Your plans must accept written requests in all cases, but may accept oral requests for standard cases. In the case of expedited coverage requests, the plan must accept oral requests for expedited coverage determinations and expedited re-determinations.

Approved exceptions are valid for prescription refills for the remainder of the plan year, as long as you remain in the plan, your doctor continues to prescribe the drug, and the drug remains safe for your condition. Your doctor determines if the drug continues to be safe for your condition.

At the end of the plan year, the plan will notify members of coverage for the following year. During the Annual Coordinated Election Period is when you need to consider switching to another drug. An appeal that is effective is only good for the balance of the year in which it is approved. Also, it is only approved for the number of prescription refills that you have remaining with the prescription. Do you want to have to go through this process every year? I doubt it. So, you may want to switch plans when you can for the next year.

Unlike the approved exception process, which is valid for the balance of the year, a prior authorization approval may not be valid for that long. Here, the prior authorization is provided for only the number of prescription refills that you have remaining and not necessarily for the balance of the year! Again, you may not want to go through this hassle each and every year. It will be easier for you to find a plan that covers your drugs without all of the red tape.

Other Considerations

CMS has informed Part D plans to not change their illness (therapeutic) categories and classes in a formulary other than at the beginning of each plan year, except to account for new therapeutic uses and newly approved Part D drugs. A plan year is a calendar year, January through December.

After March 1, 2006, Part D plans could make maintenance changes to their formularies, such as replacing brand-name with new generic drugs or modifying formularies as a result of new information on drug safety or effectiveness. Those changes must be made in accordance with the prescribed approval procedures and following 60 days notice to all affected parties.

Part D plans are not required to obtain CMS approval or give 60 days notice when removing formulary drugs that have been withdrawn from the market by either the FDA or a product manufacturer. Please also note that beginning

At the end of the plan year, the plan will notify members of coverage for the following year. During the Annual Coordinated Election Period is when you need to consider switching to another drug.

Choosing a Medicare Part D Insurance Drug Plan

January 1, 2007, Medicare will no longer cover prescription drugs used to treat erectile dysfunction. Medicaid was prohibited from covering erectile dysfunction drugs effective January 1, 2006.

You Can Apply for Extra Help At Any Time

You may already be enrolled in a Medicare drug plan and you find out that you are eligible for the extra help Medicare offers to some people. You can apply for the extra help at any time. You can also reapply if your circumstances change. When you are already enrolled in a Medicare drug plan and you are found to be eligible for the extra help, your prescription drug plan is notified by Medicare. You do not have to be the one who notifies the plan. The plan must refund your premiums and cost-sharing assistance that you should not have paid. This goes back to the month you were found to be eligible.

How does CMS know about all of this? Well, CMS uses data submitted by state Medicaid agencies to identify people with Medicare who become entitled to full Medicaid benefits. This means you automatically qualify for extra help. If you are not in a prescription drug plan, CMS will automatically enroll you in one. Your enrollment will be effective back to the first month you were eligible for both Medicare and Medicaid (but no earlier than January 1, 2006.) You will receive this automatic enrollment notice with the name of the plan assigned to you. However, please know that you have the option to choose your own plan prior to being automatically enrolled. As long as you remain entitled to Medicare and full Medicaid benefits, you can switch plans at any time, with the new plan being effective for you starting the first of the following month.

CMS will also be notified by the state Medicaid agencies of people who become eligible for a Medicare Savings Program. These individuals will be facilitated into a plan if not already in one. The plan will be effective two months after the month CMS receives notice of their eligibility. When they receive the notice of plan assignment from CMS, they have the option to choose their own plan prior to the facilitated enrollment. Like dual eligible individuals, they can switch plans at any time, with the new plan effective the first of the following month.

Starting in spring 2005, CMS began determining individuals eligible for extra help for all of 2006. Starting in August 2006, CMS re-determined individuals for calendar year 2007 on the basis of their continued eligibility. These changes will be effective January 1, 2007. People who are currently automatically eligible for 2006 will continue to qualify for the extra help through December 2006. If you are no longer eligible, your automatic status ended on December 31, 2006.

Special Enrollment Periods

There are a number of situations when people have a Special Enrollment Period (SEP) and can add, change, or drop Medicare drug coverage. People who involuntarily lose their creditable prescription drug coverage have 60 days from the date of termination or notice of termination, whichever is later, to enroll in a Medicare drug plan. Creditable drug coverage is coverage that is as good as Medicare prescription drug coverage. People who get Medicare and Medicaid benefits (i.e., dual eligibles) or help from their state paying for their Medicare premiums (Medicare Savings Programs) may enroll in a Part D plan or switch plans at any time, with the new plan effective the first day of the following month. People who lose dual eligibility status have three months to change their Part D plan. People who permanently move out of a coverage service area for a plan have up to two months after moving to enroll in a new Part D plan. People who move into a long-term care facility, such as a nursing home, can enroll in or change plans at any time, with the new plan effective the first day of the following month. They also have two months after moving out to enroll in or change plans. People who are eligible for the extra help and were facilitated into a Part D plan have at least one opportunity to switch out of that plan during the plan year. People found eligible for the extra help after May 15, 2006, may enroll in a plan through December 31, 2006, using a Special Enrollment Period.

Coordinated Election Period

All people with Medicare can join, switch, or drop Medicare drug plans during the Annual Coordinated Election Period (AEP). The next AEP will be November 15 through December 31, 2007. Changes will be effective starting January 1, 2008 for people enrolling during this period.

There will be an AEP from November 15 through December 31 every year, with changes effective the following January 1. Each year, both stand-alone prescription drug plans (PDPs) and Medicare Advantage plans with prescription drug coverage (MA-PDs) are required to send an annual notice of change to all plan members. In 2007, the letter must be sent, along with a Summary of Benefits and a copy of the formulary for the upcoming year, in time to arrive no later than October 31, 2007. The letter will explain any changes to their current plan, including changes to the monthly premium and cost-sharing information such as co-payments or coinsurance.

In addition to the Initial Enrollment Period for Part D, and the Annual Coordinated Election Period each year, people with Medicare can join a Medicare Advantage Plan during an open enrollment period each year. People can join a new plan or switch plans. (Note that Other Medicare Plans follow different rules.)

- In 2006, the Open Enrollment Period was January 1 through June 30
- In 2007 and every year after, the Open Enrollment Period will be January 1 through March 31.
- Changes will be effective the first of the month after the person joined or switched plans

The MA Open Enrollment Period can be used to switch to a different type of plan, but it cannot be used to change whether or not the person is enrolled in Medicare prescription drug coverage.

Figure 4–2 indicates the actions you can take to change plans during the open enrollment periods (OEP) each year.

Medicare Advantage Special Plans for Special Needs Individuals

New programs Medicare now offers are specialized Medicare Advantage plans, called Special Needs Plans (5). Medicare established a Medicare Advantage (MA) option for private plans that exclusively or disproportionately enroll "special needs" individuals which are the institutionalized and people with both Medicare and Medicaid coverage. Those with severe or disabling chronic conditions would also be considered

If your coverage below is:	You can use the Open Enrollment Period (OEP) to obtain:	You CANNOT use the Open Enrollment Period (OEP) to obtain:
Medicare Advantage with prescription drug coverage	• Medicare Advantage with prescription drug coverage (MA-PD) • Original Medicare and Stand alone Prescription Drug Plan Coverage	• Medicare Advantage Prescription Drug coverage • Original Medicare and Prescription Drug Plan Coverage
Original Medicare and coverage with a prescription drug plan	• Medicare Advantage with prescription drug coverage (MA-PD)	
Original Medicare Only	• Medicare Advantage Only	• Medicare Advantage Prescription Drug Coverage • Original Medicare and Prescription Drug Plan Coverage

Adapted from Medicare & You, p. 65, Centers for Medicare and Medicaid Services

Figure 4–2   Medicare Advantage Open Enrollment Period Limits
Source: Adapted from Medicare & You, p. 65, Centers for Medicare and Medicaid Services.

a "special needs" group, such as people with diabetes, congestive heart failure, mental illness, or HIV/AIDS. End-Stage Renal Disease (ESRD) eligible individuals would be another example of a "special needs" group. (Previously ESRD-eligible individuals could not enroll in a Medicare Advantage plan, unless they were already enrolled and developed ESRD after enrollment.) These specialized MA plans will be paid on the same basis as other Medicare Advantage Plans and will be available for periods before January 1, 2009.

Changes in the Standard Benefit for 2007 (6)

See Figure 4–3 for a depiction of what these changes will look like. The standard benefit is the minimum coverage plans must provide. The limits will increase in 2007 as follows:

- Your deductible goes from $250 in 2006 to $265 in 2007
- The initial coverage limit moves from $2,250 to $2,400 in 2007
- The out-of-pocket expense amount moves from $3,600 in 2006 to $3,850 in 2007
- The total out-of-pocket cost amount moves from $5,100 in 2006 to $5,451.25 in 2007
- Your minimum cost-sharing in the catastrophic coverage goes from $2 in 2006 to $2.15 in 2007 for generic or preferred drugs and from $5.00 in 2006 to $5.35 in 2007 for all other drugs. Your pharmacist can help you know what the specific drugs are for you.
- People with dual eligibility, Medicare, and full Medicaid benefits (full-benefit dual eligible individuals) who are in nursing homes continue to pay nothing for Medicare-covered drugs
- The maximum co-payments below the out-of-pocket threshold for full-benefit dual-eligible people with incomes up to 100% of the Federal poverty level are $1 for generic or preferred drugs (no change from 2006) and $3.10 (up from $3.00) for all other drugs in 2007

- Other people eligible for the extra help (LIS = limited income subsidy) will pay $2.15 (up from $2.00) for generic/preferred drugs and $5.35 (up from $5.00) for all other drugs

In addition, people who receive the partial subsidy will pay a $53.00 annual deductible (up from $50 in 2006) and will continue to pay cost-sharing of 15%.

True Out of Pocket (TrOOP) Costs

Under the defined standard benefit in 2006, the coverage gap—for plans that have one—begins after people reach $2,250 in total drug costs. This is called the initial coverage limit, and includes the total cost of the drug, not just the person's "true out-of-pocket" (TrOOP) costs.

After reaching the initial coverage limit, people pay 100% of their drug costs in the gap until their TrOOP costs total $3,600. Once people spend $3,600 out-of-pocket for covered

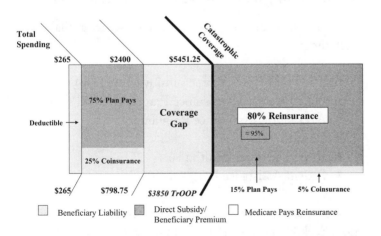

Standard Benefit 2007

Figure 4–3   Standard Benefit 2007
Source: www.medicare.gov.

Choosing a Medicare Part D Insurance Drug Plan

drug costs during the year, they pay 5% (or a small co-payment of $2 for generic or preferred drugs and $5 for all other drugs) for the rest of the calendar year. This is called catastrophic coverage, and it could start even sooner in some plans. These amounts will change each year.

Payments that will count toward a your true out-of-pocket (TrOOP) costs include those made by

- You the plan member
- Your family members or other individuals
- State pharmacy assistance programs (PAPs)
- Any extra help (low-income subsidy)
- Charities
  - Unless established, run, or controlled by a current or former employer or union
  - May include Patient Assistance Programs (PAPs), including manufacturer-sponsored PAPs, if established as a charity to help pay cost-sharing

As noted the true out of pocket (TrOOP) cost limits will increase during 2007.

What Else Might I Do to See What Is Available for Me?

In addition, people can explore other assistance available (6), including:

- The Part D low-income subsidy (extra help)
- State Pharmacy Assistance Programs (SPAPs)
- AIDS Drug Assistance Programs
- Charities
- Employer/group health plans
- Patient Assistance Programs (PAPs)

Above all else, know that this is very complicated information. Seek help early and often to make this work for you in the very best way possible!

References

1. *Comparing Medicare Prescription Drug Coverage.* United States Public Health Service, Centers for Medicare and Medicaid Services, CMS Publication Number 11110, June, 2006.
2. Freking, Kevin. Medicare error sends checks to thousands, *Wichita Eagle*: www.kansas.com/mld/kansas/news/nation/15336346.htm accessed 23 August 2006
3. *Medicare & You, 2006.* United States Public Health Service, Centers for Medicare and Medicaid Services, CMS Publication Number 10050, January, 2006.
4. Medicare Prescription Drug, Improvement, and Modernization Act of 2003, Section 231; www.medicare.gov
5. www.cms.hhs.gov/SpecialNeedsPlans/
6. www.kff.org/medicare/index.cfm Kaiser Family Foundation, Medicare, site accessed August 20, 2006.

CHAPTER 5

What Drugs Are Covered?

Drugs for All Diseases and Ailments—but not All Drugs

The Medicare Part D drug benefit provides for the use of drugs from drug classes treating virtually all diseases and ailments. CMS has worked with outside groups to develop what is termed a model formulary. This means that each of the prescription drug plans and Medicare Advantage plans that have a drug program must meet general guidelines for formularies. In effect, this means that you should have access to medications in every class of drugs available. Again let me stress that your particular drugs may not be on the formulary of your plan. This is why it is so important to check all of this out before you enroll in a specific plan. If for some reason, you are not satisfied with the plan that you have chosen for the year, you can change plans. You will have to wait until the end of the year to do so.

There are 146 different drug classes and categories for which drugs in these classes must be offered to you. CMS has indicated that they will periodically check these formularies against the standards that they have set for the drug formulary system. The only way to be sure your drugs are covered is to check and make sure.

Drugs Covered in the Model Formulary Guidelines

The most commonly prescribed drugs are contained in the formularies that CMS approves for the prescription drug plans and Medicare Advantage plans. Examples of the types of drugs include (this is not a complete listing):

Type of Drug	What the drug is used to treat
Analgesics	Drugs for pain
Antibiotics	Drugs for infections
Seizure drugs	Drugs taken to prevent epileptic seizures
Drugs for dementia	Drugs to help conditions such as Alzheimer's Disease
Antidepressants	Drugs to help control depression
Alcohol deterrents	Drug such as disulfiram (Antabuse$^®$)
Anti-emetics	Drugs taken to prevent or diminish nausea, taken with cancer drugs
Antifungals	Drugs taken to control fungal infections
Antigout	Drugs taken to lower uric acid and help to control gout attacks
Arthritis drugs	These drugs are called non-steroidal anti-inflammatory drugs (NSAIDS) are taken to help control arthritis
Anti-migraine drugs	Drugs to impact migraine headaches
Cancer drugs	Antineoplastic drugs
Antiparasitic drugs	Drugs taken to affect parasite infections
Drugs for Parkinson's Disease	Antiparkinson drugs
Antipsychotic drugs	Drugs used to treat mental disorders
Antiviral drugs	Drugs to treat viral infections

Type of Drug	What the drug is used to treat
Bipolar drugs	Drugs to treat manic depressive disorder
Blood glucose regulators	These drugs can either be injected drugs—insulin, or oral agents to control diabetes—oral hypoglycemic agents
Cardiovascular drugs	Drugs for heart failure—such as digoxin
	Drugs for high blood pressure— beta blockers, alpha blockers, alpha agonists, antiarrhythmias, calcium channel blockers, ACE inhibitors, ARBs, diuretics
Blood cholesterol drugs	Drugs to lower cholesterol, lipid levels, triglycerides
Dental or oral agents	Drugs such as antibiotics taken to treat gingivitis or to prevent it from occurring
Stomach drugs	Various gastrointestinal drugs
Drugs for enlarged prostate	Benign prostatic hypertrophy drugs
Drugs to lower inflammation	These drugs are called glucocorticoid drugs, they are steroids
Drugs for osteoporosis	These are drugs taken daily or in some cases once a month
Female hormones	Estrogens or progestins
Vaccines	Vaccines such as pneuomococcal pneumonia vaccine
Eye drops	Ophthalmic drugs to treat various eye disorders such as glaucoma
Otic drops	Drugs for us in the ear
Breathing drugs	Drugs used to treat various lung ailments

What Drugs Are Covered?

Type of Drug	What the drug is used to treat
Drugs for sleep	Drugs used to help you sleep at night
Muscle relaxants	Drugs to treat skeletal muscle problems
Prenatal vitamins	These are the only vitamins Medicare Part D will pay for

These are just some of the drugs that are covered in these formularies that Medicare requires drug plans to maintain.

How to Find Out What Drugs the Prescription Drug Plans Will Pay for

Formulary finder. Figure 5–1 shows the CMS website tool available to you to find prescription drug plans available to you where you live. Initially click on the Formulary Finder tab. After you click on the State where you live, you can then begin to enter the drugs that you take. The example below lists the drug—Coreg®. You then enter the remaining drugs that you take. You will be notified if there is a generic available or not. You can keep adding more drugs that you take until you have entered each drug. Then you simply touch the "continue with existing drugs" option. You will then see the prescription drug plans in your State that have the drugs that you entered on the formulary of the plan. You should examine these plans carefully to determine which ones have the most coverage of your drugs, and then see what the specifics of the plan are concerning premiums and coverage in the "donut hole" gap.

Here you will begin to list the drugs that you currently are taking, and you can then find out which plans in your area provide the greatest number of drugs that you take on the formulary for the prescription drug plan. As previously noted, the drugs are entered one at a time until all that you are taking have been entered. At this point, the 'continue with these drugs' tab is clicked.

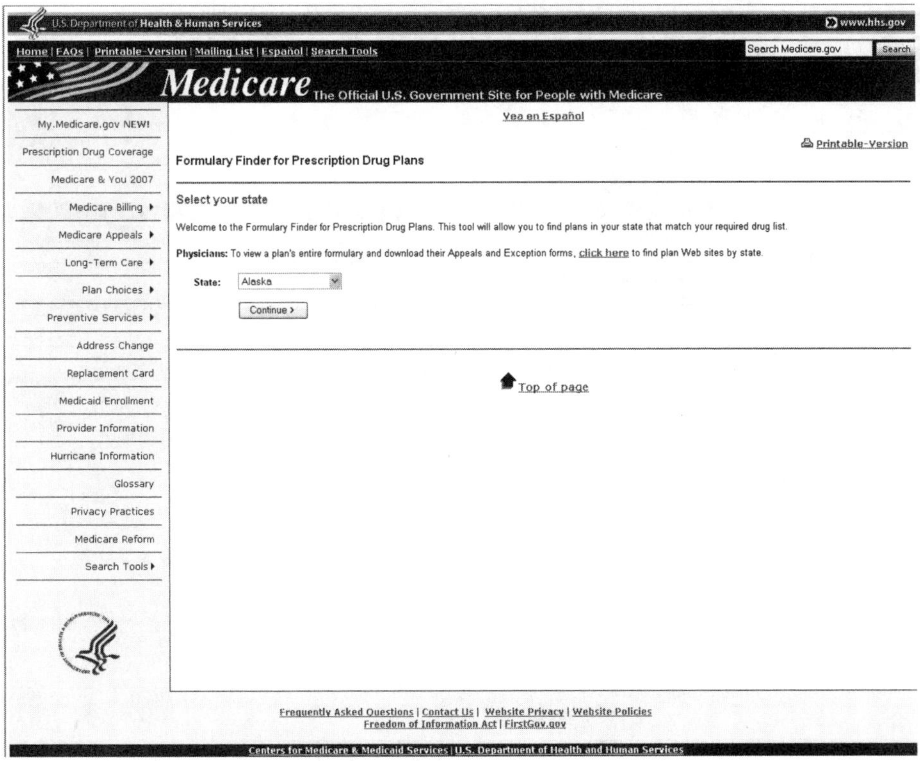

Figure 5–1   Formulary Finder 1st Page
Source: http://formularyfinder.medicare.gov/formularyfinder/selectstate.asp

Once all the drugs have been entered, you then are presented with the prescription drug plans in your state that cover the drugs that you take. There is also a column (the 4th one) that lists the number of pharmacies in the state that participate in the plan and provides coverage for your drugs. The more pharmacies that are listed, the more extensive the coverage is for you. This is a good indicator of the ease in which you will be able to obtain your medications.

Please ask for help if you have trouble navigating through the websites that inform you about the prescription drug plans. This is a confusing program with many complex parts. Use resources that you have available to get help to benefit the most that you can.

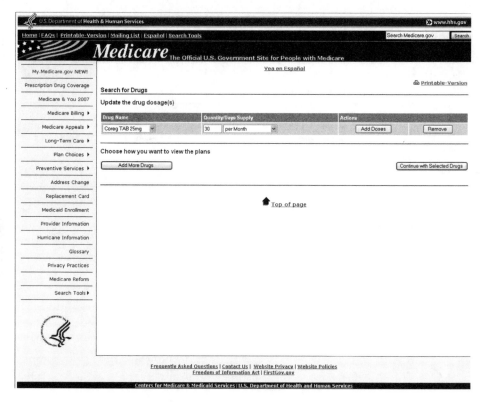

Figure 5–2   Formulary Finder 2nd Page, enter Coreg
Source: http://formularyfinder.medicare.gov/formularyfinder/drugSelect.asp?vid=175573707
&cmbState=AK&plan_specific=False&language=English&StyleChoice_Size=0&alpha_search=fa
lse#searchBox

Coverage for Drugs Under Medicare Part B

Next, let me describe the drugs that are still available under
previous Medicare coverage. This is Medicare Part B. There
are some drugs that are covered under Medicare Part B that
can be seen in the following chart provided by the United
States Agency on Aging (see Figure 5–6). The source is the
Agency on Aging website: www.aoa.gov/Medicare/re-
sources/PartsBDFeb6finaldraftV6.doc.

Some of these drugs covered under Medicare Part B fall
under the durable medical equipment (DME) portion of
Medicare. Medicare Part B generally will cover a limited set

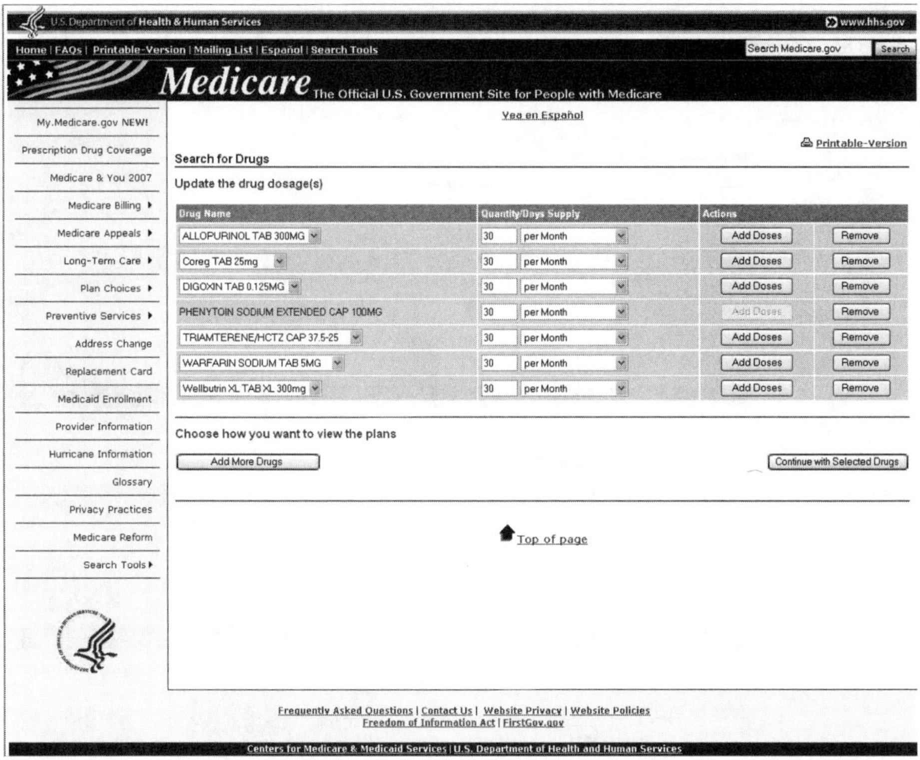

Figure 5–3   Formulary Finder 3rd Page
Source: http://formularyfinder.medicare.gov/formularyfinder/drugSelectRefine.asp?vid=
175568435&cmbState=&plan_Specific=&language=&styleChoice_Size=&seGenerics=true

of prescription drugs. Medicare Part B covers injectable and infusible drugs that are not usually self-administered and that are furnished and administered as part of a physician service. If the injection is usually self-administered (e.g., Imitrex®) or is not furnished and administered as part of a physician service, it may not be covered by Part B but will be covered under Medicare Part D. I would encourage you to work with your doctor and pharmacist to find the best coverage options for your drugs covered by these two parts of Medicare.

If Medicare Part A or Part B pays for drugs as prescribed and dispensed or administered, that drug cannot be covered for that person under Part D. The person may have to pay the deductible under Part B.

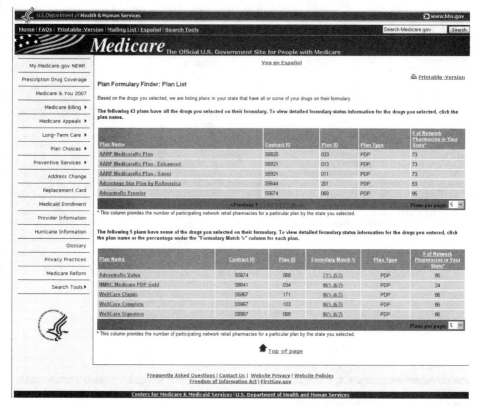

Figure 5–4   Formulary Finder 4th Page
Source: http://formularyfinder.medicare.gov/formularyfinder/drugSelect.asp?vid=175570521&cmb
State=AK&plan_specific=False&language=English&StyleChoice_Size=0&alpha_search=false#
searchBox

Non-covered Drugs in Any Formulary

There are several types of drugs that are *not* available for coverage in the Medicare Part D program. These drug classes include:

- Over-the-counter drugs
- Barbiturates
- Benzodiazepines
- Vitamins

It does not matter if your doctor has written you prescriptions for these drugs. They are not covered under Medicare Part D.

Medicare Parts B/D Coverage Issues

This table provides a quick reference guide for the most frequent Medicare Part B drug and Part D drug coverage determination scenarios facing Part D plans and Part D pharmacy providers. It does not address all possible situations. For a more extensive discussion, please refer to "Medicare Part B vs. Part D Coverage Issues" at http://www.cms.hhs.gov/PrescriptionDrugCovGenIn/Downloads/PartBandPartDdoc_07.27.05.pdf.

Part B Coverage Category	Part B Coverage Description	If Retail Pharmacy, Which Part Pays?[1]	If LTC Pharmacy, Which Part Pays?	Comments
Durable Medical Equipment (DME) Supply Drugs **Only available for people living at "home"**[2]	Drugs that require administration via covered DME (e.g., inhalation drugs requiring a nebulizer, IV drugs "requiring"[3] a pump for infusion, insulin via infusion pump)[4]	**B**	**D**	Blood glucose testing strips and lancets covered under Part B DME benefit are never available under Part D because they are not Part D drugs.
Drugs furnished "incident to" a physician service (i.e., the drug is furnished by the physician and administered either by the physician or by the physician's staff under the physician's supervision).	Injectable/intravenous drugs 1) administered incident to a physician service and 2) considered by Part B carrier as "not usually self-administered"	**D**	**D**	Not covered by Part B because a pharmacy cannot provide a drug incident to a physician's service (i.e., only a physician office would bill Part B for "incident to" drugs).
Immunosuppressant Drugs	Drugs used in immunosuppressive therapy for people who received transplant from Medicare-approved facility and were entitled to Medicare Part A at time of transplant (i.e., "Medicare-Covered Transplant")	**B or D:** **Part B** for Medicare-Covered Transplant **Part D** for all other situations	**B or D:** **Part B** for Medicare-Covered Transplant **Part D** for all other situations	Participating Part B pharmacies must bill the DMERC in their region when these drugs are covered under Part B.
Oral Anti-Cancer Drugs	Oral drugs used for cancer treatment that contain same active ingredient (or pro-drug) as injectable dosage forms that would be covered as 1) not usually self-administered and 2) provided incident to a physician's service	**B or D:** **Part B** for cancer treatment **Part D** for all other indications	**B or D:** **Part B** for cancer treatment **Part D** for all other indications	Participating Part B pharmacies must bill the DMERC in their region when these drugs are covered under Part B.
Oral Anti-emetic Drugs	Oral anti-emetic drugs used as full therapeutic replacement for IV anti-emetic drugs within 48 hrs of chemo	**B or D:** **Part B** for use w/in 48 hrs. of chemo **Part D** all other situations	**B or D:** **Part B** for use w/in 48 hrs. of chemo **Part D** all other situations	Participating Part B pharmacies must bill the DMERC in their region when these drugs are covered under Part B.
Erythropoietin (EPO)	Treatment of anemia for persons with chronic renal failure who are undergoing dialysis	**B or D:** **Part B** for treatment of anemia for people undergoing dialysis **Part D** all other situations	**B or D:** **Part B** for treatment of anemia for people undergoing dialysis **Part D** all other situations	EPO may also be covered under Part B for other conditions if furnished incident to a physician's service. (A physician, not a pharmacy, bills for "incident to" drugs.)
Prophylactic Vaccines	Influenza; Pneumococcal; and Hepatitis B (for intermediate to high-risk individuals)	**B or D:** **Part B** for Influenza, Pneumococcal, & Hepatitis B (for intermediate to high risk) **Part D** for all others	**B or D:** **Part B** for influenza, pneumococcal, & Hepatitis B (for intermediate to high risk) **Part D** for all others	Vaccines given directly related to the treatment of an injury or direct exposure to a disease or condition are always covered under Part B.
Parenteral Nutrition	Prosthetic benefit for individuals with "permanent" dysfunction of the digestive tract (must meet "permanence" test)	**B or D:** **Part B** if "permanent" dysfunction of digestive tract **Part D** for all other situations	**B or D:** **Part B** if "permanent" dysfunction of digestive tract **Part D** for all other situations	Part D does not pay for the equipment/supplies and professional services associated with the provision of parenteral nutrition or other Part D covered infusion therapy.

Figure 5–5   Formulary Finder 5th Page

Source: http://formularyfinder.medicare.gov/formularyfinder/drugSelectRefine.asp?vid=175570521&cmbState=AK&plan_specific=&language=&StyleChoice_Size&useGenerics=true

What Drugs Are Covered?

Medicare Parts B/D Coverage Issues

This table provides a quick reference guide for the most frequent Medicare Part B drug and Part D drug coverage determination scenarios facing Part D plans and Part D pharmacy providers. It does not address all possible situations. For a more extensive discussion, please refer to "Medica Part B vs. Part D Coverage Issues" at http://www.cms.hhs.gov/PrescriptionDrugCovGenIn/Downloads/PartBandPartDdoc_07.27.05.pdf.

Part B Coverage Category	Part B Coverage Description	If Retail Pharmacy, Which Part Pays?[1]	If LTC Pharmacy, Which Part Pays?	Comments
Durable Medical Equipment (DME) Supply Drugs **Only available for people living at "home"[2]**	Drugs that require administration via covered DME (e.g., inhalation drugs requiring a nebulizer, IV drugs "requiring"[3] a pump for infusion, insulin via infusion pump)[4]	B	D	Blood glucose testing strips and lancets covered under Part B DME benefit are never available under Part D because they are not Part D drugs.
Drugs furnished "incident to" a physician service (i.e., the drug is furnished by the physician and administered either by the physician or by the physician's staff under the physician's supervision).	Injectable/intravenous drugs 1) administered incident to a physician service and 2) considered by Part B carrier as "not usually self-administered"	D	D	Not covered by Part B because a pharmacy cannot provide a drug incident to a physician's service (i.e., only a physician office would bill Part B for "incident to" drugs).
Immunosuppressant Drugs	Drugs used in immunosuppressive therapy for people who received transplant from Medicare-approved facility and were entitled to Medicare Part A at time of transplant (i.e., "Medicare-Covered Transplant")	**B or D:** Part B for Medicare-Covered Transplant **Part D** for all other situations	**B or D:** Part B for Medicare-Covered Transplant **Part D** for all other situations	Participating Part B pharmacies must bill the DMERC in their region when these drugs are covered under Part B.
Oral Anti-Cancer Drugs	Oral drugs used for cancer treatment that contain same active ingredient (or pro-drug) as injectable dosage forms that would be covered as 1) not usually self-administered and 2) provided incident to a physician's service	**B or D:** Part B for cancer treatment **Part D** for all other indications	**B or D:** Part B for cancer treatment **Part D** for all other indications	Participating Part B pharmacies must bill the DMERC in their region when these drugs are covered under Part B.
Oral Anti-emetic Drugs	Oral anti-emetic drugs used as full therapeutic replacement for IV anti-emetic drugs within 48 hrs of chemo	**B or D:** Part B for use w/in 48 hrs. of chemo **Part D** all other situations	**B or D:** Part B for use w/in 48 hrs. of chemo **Part D** all other situations	Participating Part B pharmacies must bill the DMERC in their region when these drugs are covered under Part B.
Erythropoietin (EPO)	Treatment of anemia for persons with chronic renal failure who are undergoing dialysis	**B or D:** Part B for treatment of anemia for people undergoing dialysis **Part D** all other situations	**B or D:** Part B for treatment of anemia for people undergoing dialysis **Part D** all other situations	EPO may also be covered under Part B for other conditions if furnished incident to a physician's service. (A physician, not a pharmacy, bills for "incident to" drugs.)
Prophylactic Vaccines	Influenza; Pneumococcal; and Hepatitis B (for intermediate to high-risk individuals)	**B or D:** Part B for Influenza, Pneumococcal, & Hepatitis B (for intermediate to high risk) **Part D** for all others	**B or D:** Part B for influenza, pneumococcal, & Hepatitis B (for intermediate to high risk) **Part D** for all others	Vaccines given directly related to the treatment of an injury or direct exposure to a disease or condition are always covered under Part B.
Parenteral Nutrition	Prosthetic benefit for individuals with "permanent" dysfunction of the digestive tract (must meet "permanence" test)	**B or D:** Part B if "permanent" dysfunction of digestive tract **Part D** for all other situations	**B or D:** Part B if "permanent" dysfunction of digestive tract **Part D** for all other situations	Part D does not pay for the equipment/supplies and professional services associated with the provision of parenteral nutrition or other Part D covered infusion therapy.

Figure 5–6   Medicare Parts B/D Coverage Issues

Source: www.aoa.gov/Medicare/resources/PartsBDFeb6finaldraftV6.doc

Over-the-counter drugs (OTC) (This is not a complete listing). OTC drugs include products such as aspirin (Bayer® and many other brands), acetaminophen (Tylenol® and many other brands), ibuprofen (Motrin®, Advil®, or many other brands), naproxen (Aleve® or many other brands), omeprazole (Prilosec OTC®), famotidine (Pepcid AC® or many other brands), ranitidine (Zantac® or many other brands), and/or milk of magnesia (Phillips® or many other brands).

Barbiturates. These include many differing types of products that may include phenobarbital, secobarbital, pentobarbital, and others.

Benzodiazepines. These drugs may include Ativan® (lorazepam), Centrax® (prazepam), Dalmane® (flurazepam), Librium® (chlordiazepoxide), Restaril® (temazepam), Tranxene® (chlorazepate dipotassium), Serax® (oxazepam), Halcion® (triazolam), Valium® (diazepam), Xanax® (alprazolam), etc.

Vitamins. These can be multivitamins (vitamin and mineral combinations in one tablet) or individual vitamins separately. Some examples are Vitamin C, individual Vitamin B supplements [any number of Vitamin Bs: B_1, B_2, B_5 (niacin), B_6, or B_{12}], Vitamin E, or other supplements containing vitamins or minerals. Minerals can include iron supplements, calcium tablets, or calcium with Vitamin D.

Technically, insulin is a non-prescription product, but insulin is covered under Medicare Part D if it has been prescribed by your doctor.

I hope this chapter has provided you with some tips to use when considering the drugs that are and are not covered by the Medicare Part D prescription drug programs. The bottom line here is that it is really important to know in general what the program will pay for (therapeutic categories), and to have what drugs will not be covered (e.g., over-the-counter drugs or some types of prescription medications). This is very confusing information, please ask your pharmacist to help you understand the difference between the varying categories of drugs.

CHAPTER 6

How to Choose a Pharmacist

The Importance of Your Pharmacist

The pharmacist that you choose to fill your prescriptions for any prescription, but especially for Medicare Part D prescriptions, will play a key role in helping you with your medications and questions about them and about Medicare. Many times we spend a great deal of time selecting the right person to take care of our needs. We spend a great deal of time finding just the right car mechanics, home repair persons, bankers, and others that perform important functions in our lives. You should spend even more time selecting your pharmacist. Outside of your physicians, your pharmacist can provide you with more significant therapeutic drug information than any other health professional. But with Medicare Part D, choosing your pharmacist is even more important. It is very important to choose your pharmacist well, and examine what is important to you as a patient as you seek care and information from a pharmacist.

It is important in Medicare Part D to choose your pharmacist carefully. Let them help you as much as possible!

Referrals from Friends

Your friends and acquaintances are good sources of information about pharmacies. If someone you know has had good luck with a pharmacy, chances are good that you will as well. Check with those you know and know well regarding how

The pharmacist is some-
one you need to be able
to rely upon not just for
Medicare Part D ques-
tions, but other health
related information as
well.

they are treated at their pharmacy. Do they feel comfortable recommending their pharmacist to you? Are the services that they receive equally important to you? Do they trust their pharmacist and pharmacy to take care of all their medication needs? People will be honest with you, and I certainly encourage you to ask people you trust to give you their advice. The pharmacist is someone you need to be able to rely upon not just for Medicare Part D questions, but other health related information as well. Be sure to ask the pharmacist what services are provided in the pharmacy.

Is the Pharmacist Accessible?

Pharmacists are the most accessible health professional, and you should use them to the fullest extent possible. In fact, your pharmacist needs to be readily accessible to you for your needs concerning the medications that you are taking. Your pharmacist can be an invaluable source of information about drugs, their effects, and proper usage. You should be able to ask your pharmacist about side effects, adverse reactions, and expectations for your drug therapy. There is no one in the health care system who is as knowledgeable about drugs, and is as approachable in the practice setting as a pharmacist.

You should be able to ask your pharmacist a question at anytime about any of the medications that you currently take or are considering taking. If you are unsure who you are speaking with at the pharmacy, always ask to speak with the pharmacist. If the pharmacist responds that "this is not a good time to talk," find a time that would be acceptable to you both. Set a time to talk later about your questions and concerns.

Your pharmacist cannot tell you which prescription drug plan to choose, or steer you toward one plan over another. However, the pharmacist can help you determine the exact names and spellings for the drugs that you take. The pharmacist can also let you know if a generic equivalent is available for some of the drugs that you currently have been prescribed. The amount of money that you spend over the course of a year can also be projected with the help of a pharmacist. These are important pieces of information that you must have when deciding on a Medicare Part D Plan. With this preliminary information, you are then in a position to make choices about a plan that is best for you. It takes time to go through the plans in your area to determine which is best for you. It takes me about an hour per person to go through drugs that are taken, which plan might be best for a person, and how to go about helping them make the best choice for their needs.

Your pharmacist cannot tell you which Medicare Part D prescription drug plan to choose, or steer you toward one plan over another.

Can I Call for More Information and Speak to the Pharmacist Every Time?

It may be that you can speak with the pharmacist on the phone and receive the answers that you seek. Pharmacists are very accustomed to speaking with doctors, nurses, and patients on the phone. It is commonplace, and is a good way for you to ensure privacy and obtain the information that is needed. You may have more time to talk on the phone with the pharmacist than in a face to face scenario. Find out what works best for you and your needs, and follow through to find the answers you are seeking.

Find a time when it is best for you and for your pharmacist to answer questions about Medicare Part D.

General Concerns About Drugs and Drug Use

There are several things to think about when you choose a pharmacist to provide you with the drugs that you take, and the information for you that needs to accompany the prescriptions. Always ask those that provide care for you if you need to continue to take the drugs that you currently take. It may be that you can discontinue one or more drugs. Always check with your physician and pharmacist before you start to take an additional drug, or discontinue a drug you take now.

Concerns About Certain Medications If You Are Caring for an Elderly Individual

Researchers have compiled lists of 66 drugs considered unsafe for use in the elderly.[1] Make sure that your pharmacist

How to Choose a Pharmacist

knows about this list, the drugs that are on the list, and can supply you with suggested treatment alternatives. There are numerous sources that present this type of information, and your pharmacist should know where to look in order to obtain the information.

Counseling When Obtaining New Prescriptions

Always check with your physician and pharmacist before you start to take an additional drug, or discontinue a drug you take now.

Pharmacists routinely provide important information to patients about the drugs they are prescribed. This is called patient counseling. United States federal law, and subsequent state rules and regulations, require that you are offered counseling on prescriptions that you have filled. These federal regulations (Omnibus Budget Reconciliation Act of 1990) [OBRA '90] were initially applicable to patients receiving care through the various State Medicaid assistance programs, however, all states have now passed regulations that expand this requirement to all patients.

The offer of counseling means just that; you should be asked if you would like to hear information about your medications. Often what happens is you are asked to sign a signature log that is thrust in front of you that says you have declined the offer to receive counseling. Many people think that signing this signature book simply indicates that they have picked up a prescription, but this is not the case. You should be informed what this signature form means, and be asked if you would care to receive information about the drugs that you are receiving. The letter of the law is being met by the signature log, but this does not fulfill the pharmacist's obligation to you to counsel you if you would like to receive further information.

It is unethical for a pharmacist to refuse to speak with you about your medications. Insist that you receive instructions on proper use of the drugs prescribed and dispensed to you. If for some reason, it is not convenient for either you or the pharmacist to fully counsel you when you pick up a prescription, find a time in your schedule when it would be convenient for you to speak with the pharmacist by phone if necessary.

You do not need to wait until you have a prescription filled before asking a pharmacist about your medications. You can call and speak to your pharmacist at any time. Also, you can speak to a pharmacist if you happen to be in the pharmacy and have a question. A pharmacist should always be available to answer your questions, whether you happen to be a patient at that pharmacy or not. Virtually every pharmacist will assist you with answering questions regardless of where you obtain your medications. There are occasions when your pharmacist may be too busy to speak with you. If you continuously have trouble when trying to speak with your pharmacist, consider finding a new pharmacy.

Pharmacists can answer questions about the drugs that you take even if you obtain your prescriptions from another pharmacy.

How to Choose a Pharmacist

Brand and Generic Drugs

There are several possible types of drugs that can be dispensed for you as a patient in Medicare Part D. A drug may be available as only a brand name product. When a new drug is first on the market, there is not a generic option available to you. The prescriptions for the drug can only be filled with one particular product. In this case, the product may have a varying length of patent protection. This depends on the amount of time it took for the drug to reach the market after progressing through the required phases of approval necessary required by the United States Food and Drug Administration (FDA). A generic drug is available when the brand name drug goes "off patent" protection. Under Medicare Part D, your co-payment is less with generic drugs than it is for brand name drugs.

In order to save you money in Medicare Part D, your physician may write prescription for a generic substitute for a medication. Your pharmacist may also provide a generic substitute in order to save you money. Generic substitutes are available for some, but not all brand name prescription drugs. By asking your pharmacist if a generic is available for your prescription, you will save money. These generic drugs are safe, and I would urge you to use them when you can. They will do the same thing for you that a brand name drug will do, but they are just much less expensive. The only time I would *not* use a generic drug in place of a brand name drug is if you are take a drug called phenytoin (Dilantin®) to prevent seizures. I feel it is not safe to switch from the brand name drug Dilantin® to the generic option. However, if you are starting to take the drug for the first time, feel confident in taking the generic form right off. I feel the problems occur when switching from one to the other occurs. This drug has a distribution in the body that is important, and it needs to be the same distribution every time you take it in order to have the same effect. This lowers the possibility you might have a seizure. The medical literature contains papers that describe this situation.[2]

Charging for Services

If you are being charged extra for services over and above what you are paying for prescriptions, and have not agreed to purchase extra services, you are probably being over charged. A pharmacist may provide expanded services for you, services for which you have agreed to pay, and there is nothing wrong with this. However, if you are being charged for the pharmacist contacting your physician or insurance company on your behalf, you are being overcharged. If you are being told that you have to pay a membership fee in order to obtain services, you are being unethically treated. If you have a certain type of insurance, and you are being told by the pharmacist that you will have to pay extra in order to receive care, this is wrong. If you are told that you have to pay extra because you are asking to have your prescriptions transferred to another pharmacy, you are deceived and treated unethically by the pharmacist.

Refusal to Fill Your Prescription

Be sure to find out if your current pharmacy is in the network of providers in your Medicare Part D Plan before you sign up for the prescription drug plan.

A pharmacist may choose not to fill your prescription. That is a right that pharmacists have in some cases. Some pharmacists choose to not compound prescriptions from basic ingredients to make creams, ointments, or some liquid preparations. Some pharmacies do not participate in specific drug benefit plans; this varies and may affect some more than others. Pharmacists are not required to participate in all plans available to consumers. In fact, there may be some plans that exclude some pharmacies from participating.

It is not legal for a pharmacist to refuse to fill a prescription because of your personal characteristics. Nor is it legal to fill only certain prescriptions for certain individuals and not for others even though they both have the same drug coverage. A pharmacist cannot choose to fill some prescriptions for you because they are profitable, and choose to not fill others due to a low profit margin. If you have Medicare Part D insurance coverage for your prescription drugs, and the drug you are seeking is covered under the insurance policy, the pharmacist should fill your prescription.

There are instances when it is professionally justifiable to not fill a prescription for a patient. If a pharmacist refuses to fill a prescription due to the presence of a drug interaction with other medications you are taking, or it appears that there is an error on the part of the physician in prescribing a certain medication, there is certainly a good reason for not filling the prescription. If there appears to be overuse of certain drugs, a previous documented intolerance on the part of the patient to a drug or a class of drugs, this too is a reason for not filling a prescription. In these cases, the pharmacist is serving as the patient's advocate.

Furnishing You the Best Price Available

Always find out how much you can save with taking generic drugs in place of brand name drugs. Is there a generic equivalent available in the series of drugs in a class of drugs from which you might be taking one? If there is a generic drug available for your prescription, find out if you are eligible to receive this when filling your prescription. The pharmacist can help you with finding the answer to this question. If you are receiving a generic substitute, find out how much savings you can expect. If you pay a co-payment for your prescriptions, find out how to best maximize your payment of the co-payment. If you can obtain several months supply of a

If you have Medicare Part D insurance coverage for your prescription drugs, and the drug you are seeking is covered under the insurance policy, the pharmacist should fill your prescription. The pharmacy must be in the network of providers for the prescription drug plan.

How to Choose a Pharmacist

maintenance medication and pay just one co-payment, you will save money. The only way you will know the answers to these questions is to ask your pharmacist.

Drugs and Expiration (Freshness) Dating

All drugs are required to have a manufacturer supplied expiration date for each prescription medication marketed in the United States. Pharmacies routinely check for outdated products, and have mechanisms to return the product to the manufacturer for replacements or refunds. Most prescriptions when dispensed have, as a rule, an expiration date that is listed as one year from the date of prescription filling. However, you may be dispensed a drug with a shorter amount of shelf life available, and if this is the case, the one year date is not correct. You will not know what the original expiration date is unless you ask the pharmacist. Just make sure that the drugs that you are receiving are in date and correctly marked. Some items such as ophthalmic (for use in the eyes), or otic (for use in the ears) preparations have a shorter expiration date due to the way the items are used. For any ophthalmic preparation, I recommend that after 90 days you discard the remaining amount. You may not have to use the product for this length of time anyway. The tube or ointment may have an extended expiration date listed somewhere on the product itself. However, please note that once the sterile seal is broken as you open the product for the first time, this expiration date is invalid because the sterility of the product cannot be guaranteed. The expiration date put on these containers by the manufacturer assumes that the product is unopened and thus remains sterile, once opened the sterility is lost.

Transfer of Prescriptions from One Pharmacy to Another

It is always possible to transfer your prescription from one pharmacy to another. This assumes that the prescription in question does have refills remaining to be used. Prescriptions that are not refillable, those with no refills remaining or certain categories of prescriptions such as scheduled drugs that cannot be transferred (e.g., some pain medications and/or sleep aids) are not eligible to be transferred from one pharmacy to another. If you have your prescriptions filled at a chain pharmacy, the prescriptions can easily be transferred from one chain pharmacy location to another outlet within the same chain. This can be very handy when traveling out of state, and you are out of medications at the same time. Prescriptions filled at mail order pharmacies or local community pharmacies can also be transferred from one pharmacy to another. Do not take no for an answer if a pharmacist tells you that a prescription with refills remaining cannot be transferred from the original pharmacy to another pharmacy.

You should be able to obtain a record of the prescriptions that you have had filled at anytime you wish to see the information.

Who Owns Your Prescription?

When you have a prescription filled, the pharmacy by state law must retain the paper copy of the actual prescription. The same holds true when a physician will phone a prescription into a pharmacy for you. Having said this, you do have rights pertaining to your prescriptions. As previously noted, you do have the right to have your refillable prescriptions transferred from one pharmacy to another so as to have them filled at the new pharmacy. Pharmacies must do this if you request that they do so. You should be able to obtain a record of the prescriptions that you have had filled at anytime you wish to see the information. Pharmacies should willingly provide this information to you. If they do not do so, they are acting in an unethical manner.

Privacy and Respect

You deserve to have respect when being treated in a pharmacy. You are entitled to receive counseling from the pharmacist each and every time you have a prescription filled, or stop at the pharmacy to ask a question. Both the asking of the question and the receipt of responses should be accomplished in a quiet, private area of the pharmacy or close to it. If you do not feel comfortable with the surroundings when speaking with the pharmacist, ask to move to a more private area.

Who Are those People Back There (Filling Your Prescription)?

Behind the pharmacy counter in a retail pharmacy is the area where your prescriptions are filled and completed. There are individuals who should be there, and individual who should not be there. Pharmacy technicians are ancillary helpers who can do some of the tasks required to complete a prescription order. Technicians are allowed to retrieve bulk bottles from shelving, place the correct number of units called for on the prescription in a suitable container, and prepare a prescription label. In some states they are allowed to place a prescription label on the container, in other states they are prohibited from doing so and only the pharmacist can do this. Technicians can also prepare compounded prescriptions and intravenous (IV) preparations. The pharmacist on duty at the time of these activities then checks the work of the technician for accuracy and completeness and completes the preparation of the prescription order. In some states there are varying ratios of how many technicians can be monitored by one pharmacist. So there is variance from 1:1 technician to pharmacist ratios, or 2:1, 3:1, or 4:1 ratios allowed by varying state pharmacy rules and regulations.

Other individuals may not be present and work on prescription orders in a pharmacy. Clerks, delivery persons, or other employees are not allowed to participate in the filling of prescriptions in any state. If you suspect that this is occurring with your prescriptions when filled, contact the board of pharmacy and call the pharmacist on these activities. No one other than a pharmacist or a technician is allowed to participate in the completion of a prescription order. A pharmacist must also be present in the pharmacy when prescription orders are completed and dispensed to you.

Many states now require that pharmacists and pharmacy technicians wear nametags that indicate their status. If you cannot ascertain who is filling your prescriptions just by observation, ask probing questions until you find out who is completing your prescription orders. If in fact a non-professional individual is filling your prescription, or preparing ingredients for your prescriptions contact the pharmacist in charge in the pharmacy (they all are required to have such an individual so named) and register a complaint.

What to Do If You Suspect Something Is Not Right with How You Receive Your Prescriptions

In several of the above scenarios, I have encouraged you to be proactive regarding the prescriptions that you have filled and monitoring your pharmacy for ethical and appropriate behavior. You may have a concern about how your prescriptions are being processed. Feel free to talk with your pharmacist, or ask to see the pharmacist-in-charge (PIC). Every pharmacy has a PIC.

Virtually all pharmacies operate in an above board and ethical fashion in treating patients and families. However, since there are some who are not ethical and are breaking the law, they should be identified and reported. This is not only for your sake, but for the well-being of future patients in pharmacies. State Boards of Pharmacy are set in place to protect the health of the public; they are not set in place to protect pharmacies. So, you should consider Boards of Pharmacy to be in fact "consumer protection" agencies for your medication, health, and your family's health and well-being. If your State Board of Pharmacy does not appear to be responsive to your requests or concerns, contact the Office of the Attorney General for your state.

What If You Cannot Choose Your Pharmacy?

Because of the prescription drug plan that you belong to, you may not be able to use the pharmacy that you have used in the past. In this case, you may have to use a mail service pharmacy in order to receive coverage for your prescriptions. If

State Boards of Pharmacy are set in place to protect the health of the public; they are not set in place to protect pharmacies

If you have questions, and need to speak with a pharmacist in a mail service pharmacy, insist that you be able to speak with one when you call an 800 toll free number, or request that a pharmacist phone you at a mutually agreeable time.

How to Choose a Pharmacist

Many independent community pharmacies will not have pharmacies open for 24 hours a day, but will come back to the pharmacy to open it for emergencies.

you must use a mail order pharmacy for receiving your prescriptions because of the drug plan you have chosen, the mail order pharmacy must provide you with a toll free number to call for questions about the medications that you receive. You deserve to receive full information about medications that you take regardless of how you obtain the drugs by mail, in person, via delivery, or through someone picking up your medications and bringing them to you. If this is the case, you can still request certain things from your pharmacist, and demand that you receive them. If you have questions, and need to speak with a pharmacist in a mail service pharmacy, insist that you be able to speak with one when you call an 800 toll free number, or request that a pharmacist phone you at a mutually agreeable time.

If you need to have the pharmacy contact your physician, a mail service pharmacy can do this as well. Try to obtain the best service that you can and if for some reason the service falls short demand other options or let the decision makers who are mandating the mail option only know that you have complaints, and objectively let them know what your expectations are and how they are not being met.

Other Services

It will be useful to you to make a list of services that are important to you. Does the pharmacy deliver medications to customers' homes? Do they charge for such services? Can you fill prescriptions after hours? This may not be so important for new prescriptions, but it certainly is for refills. Many chain community pharmacies and/or food market pharmacies now have extended hours of operation, even 24 hour service, so you know that you can obtain prescriptions most anytime. But are there times even with 24 hour operations, that you may need a prescription, say on a holiday? Will there be someone who can on an emergency basis fill your prescriptions? Many independent community pharmacies will not have pharmacies open for 24 hours a day, but will come back to the pharmacy to open it for emergencies.

Because of changes in insurance coverage and specifications, you may have to have prescription medications approved before they can be filled. This is usually the case with most prescription drug plans concerning which drugs are covered under their plans. If your medication is one of these drugs, you will need what is termed "prior approval" before it can be filled. Your pharmacy can anticipate this need, contact the prescription drug plan ahead of time, and have your prescriptions ready to be filled when you need to have them filled. This is an extra, customer focused service that will save you time, and if your pharmacy provides this service, it will be very useful for you to have. These types of value added services help you realize you have made the correct choice regarding your pharmacy. If you do not have such service provided to you, you may wish to seek another pharmacy to meet you and your family's needs for pharmacy care.

The bottom line is that you must be able to trust those that provide care to you and those you care for. The once impenetrable safety net of prescription distribution in the United States has been found to be "full of holes."[3] Pharmacists have been implicated in these instances of counterfeiting and illegal distribution of fake drugs. If you do not trust those that care for you, you will not get well as you would with health professionals that you do trust. Quality, value, service, and technology (even if they are provided in an exemplary fashion) are not worth much if you cannot place trust in the providers of your health care. Trust is very important in many components of our life. It is the crucial element in relationships that you have with your health care providers including physicians, pharmacists, optometrists, podiatrists, nurses, occupational therapist, and/or physical therapists.

> Trust is very important in many components of our life. It is the crucial element in relationships that you have with your health care providers including physicians, pharmacists, optometrists, podiatrists, dieticians, nurses, occupational therapist, and/or physical therapists.

> The bottom line is that you must be able to trust those that provide care to you and those you care for.

How to Choose a Pharmacist

References

1. Fick D.M., Cooper J.W., Wade W.E. et al. Updating the Beers criteria for potentially inappropriate medication use in older adults. *Archives of Internal Medicine* 2003; 163: pp. 2716–2724.

2. Burkhardt R.T., Leppik I.E., Blesi K., Scott S, Gapany S.R. Lower phenytoin serum levels in persons switched from brand to generic phenytoin. *Neurology* 2004; 63(8): pp. 1494–6.

3. Spake A. Fake drugs, real worries: High prices and the Internet are making U.S. patients easy prey. Accessed at: http://www.usnews.com/usnews/issue/040920/health/20internet.htm, September 20, 2004.

CHAPTER 7

The Formularies In This Program and How They Work

Formularies—Definitions and Considerations

Formulary Definition

Formularies are listings of drugs that are paid for in a particular Medicare Part D Plan. These listings contain all the drugs that are eligible for a doctor to write a prescription for you that is covered by the Part D plan. Medicare defines a formulary as follows, and includes some general information about formularies as well:[1]

> "A list of drugs that a Medicare drug plan covers is called a formulary. Formularies include generic drugs and brand-name drugs. Most prescription drugs used by people with Medicare will be on a plan's formulary. The formulary must include at least two drugs in categories and classes of most commonly prescribed drugs to people with Medicare. This makes sure that people with different medical conditions can get the treatment they need."

Formulary Finder

Your physician has access to what drugs are covered by the plan you sign up for. The section is called the "Formulary Finder" and is available through www.medicare.gov. You also have the right to petition to have a certain drug that you take covered under Medicare Part D, even if a plan tells you that your drugs are not eligible for coverage. Your doctor will need to fill out part of this form. Your plan provides you with information on where this form needs to be sent. Please see Appendix D Petition Process for Formulary Addition and Notification of Non-coverage for copy of the flow of the petition once submitted. A copy of this two-page form can be found on the next page. This form has places for you and your doctor to both sign. When completed, the form will be sent to your prescription drug plan for consideration and action. Always keep copies of these types of correspondence that you send to others regarding Medicare Part D. The following page after the two-page example (Figure 7–1) shows the Medicare Part D template that plans are to use when crafting their own forms for use by enrollees.

Uncovered Drugs

There are some drugs that are not covered under Medicare Part D, even if a petition is made to have them covered. These non-covered drugs include:

- Drugs used to treat anorexia, or for weight loss or weight gain
- Drugs that are used to promote fertility
- Drugs that are used for cosmetic purposes or for hair growth
- Drugs used to treat the symptoms of a cough or cold
- Prescription vitamins or minerals, except prenatal vitamins and fluoride preparations
- Drugs that can be bought without a prescription. These are nonprescription drugs, also called over-the-counter (OTC) drugs

Plan Name _____

Phone # _____

Fax # _____

Medicare Part D Coverage Determination Request Form

This form cannot be used to request:
- Medicare non-covered drugs, including barbiturates, benzodiazepines, fertility drugs, drugs prescribed for weight loss, weight gain or hair growth, over-the-counter drugs, or prescription vitamins (except prenatal vitamins and fluoride preparations).
- Biotech or other specialty drugs for which drug-specific forms are required. [See <Part D plan website.>] OR [See links to plan websites at http://www.cms.hhs.gov/PrescriptionDrugCovGenIn/04_Formulary.asp]

Patient Information			Prescriber Information			
Patient Name:			Prescriber Name:			
Member ID#:			NPI# (if available):			
Address:			Address:			
City:	State:		City:		State:	
Home Phone:	Zip:		Office Phone #:	Office Fax #:	Zip:	
Sex (circle): M F	DOB:		Contact Person:			

Diagnosis and Medical Information		
Medication:	Strength and Route of Administration:	Frequency:
☐ New Prescription OR Date Therapy Initiated:	Expected Length of Therapy:	Qty:
Height/Weight:	Drug Allergies:	Diagnosis:
Prescriber's Signature:		Date:

Rationale for Exception Request or Prior Authorization
FORM CANNOT BE PROCESSED WITHOUT REQUIRED EXPLANATION

☐ Alternate drug(s) contraindicated or previously tried, but with adverse outcome (eg, toxicity, allergy, or therapeutic failure)

→ Specify below: (1) Drug(s) contraindicated or tried; (2) adverse outcome for each; (3) if therapeutic failure, length of therapy on each drug(s);

☐ Complex patient with one or more chronic conditions (including, for example, psychiatric condition, diabetes) is stable on current drug(s); high risk of significant adverse clinical outcome with medication change

→ Specify below: Anticipated significant adverse clinical outcome

☐ Medical need for different dosage form and/or higher dosage

→ Specify below: (1) Dosage form(s) and/or dosage(s) tried; (2) explain medical reason

☐ Request for formulary tier exception

→ Specify below: (1) Formulary or preferred drugs contraindicated or tried and failed, or tried and not as effective as requested drug; (2) if therapeutic failure, length of therapy on each drug and adverse outcome; (3) if not as effective, length of therapy on each drug and outcome

☐ Other:_____ → Explain below

REQUIRED EXPLANATION:_____

_____

Request for Expedited Review

☐ REQUEST FOR EXPEDITED REVIEW [24 HOURS]

→ BY CHECKING THIS BOX AND SIGNING ABOVE, I CERTIFY THAT APPLYING THE 72 HOUR STANDARD REVIEW TIME FRAME MAY SERIOUSLY JEOPARDIZE THE LIFE OR HEALTH OF THE MEMBER OR THE MEMBER'S ABILITY TO REGAIN MAXIMUM FUNCTION

Information on this form is protected health information and subject to all privacy and security regulations under HIPAA.

Figure 7–1   Copy of Medicare Part D Coverage Request Form Templates—page 1

Source: http://www.cms.hhs.gov/PrescriptionDrugCovGenin/Downloads;ModelCoverage DeterminationRequestForm.pdf#search=%22request%20for%20medicare%20prescription%20 drug%20coverage%20determination%22

REQUEST FOR MEDICARE PRESCRIPTION DRUG COVERAGE DETERMINATION

This form cannot be used to request barbiturates, benzodiazepines, fertility drugs, drugs for weight loss or weight gain, drugs for hair growth, over-the-counter drugs, or prescription vitamins (except prenatal vitamins and fluoride preparations)

Enrollee's/Requestor's Information

Enrollee's Name

Enrollee's Date of Birth

Enrollee's Medicare Number

Enrollee's Part D Plan ID Number

Requestor's Name (if not enrollee)

Requestor's relationship to Enrollee (attach documentation that shows authority to represent enrollee, if other than prescribing physician)

Enrollee/Requestor's Address   City   State   Zip Code

( )
Phone

Name of prescription drug you are requesting (if known, include strength, quantity and quantity requested per month):

Prescribing Physician's Information

Name

Medical Specialty

Address   City   State   Zip Code

( )   ( )
Work Phone   Fax   Office Contact Person

Type of Coverage Determination Request

☐ I need a drug that is not on the plan's list of covered drugs (formulary exception).*

☐ I have been using a drug that was previously included on the plan's list of covered drugs, but is being removed or was removed from this list during the plan year (formulary exception).*

Figure 7–1 (continued)—page 2

☐ I request an exception to the requirement that I try another drug before I get the drug my doctor prescribed (formulary exception).*

☐ I request prior authorization for the drug my doctor has prescribed.

☐ I request an exception to the plan's limit on the number of pills (quantity limit) I can receive so that I can get the number of pills my doctor prescribed (formulary exception).*

☐ My drug plan charges a higher copayment for the drug my doctor prescribed than it charges for another drug that treats my condition, and I want to pay the lower copayment (tiering exception).*

☐ I have been using a drug that was previously included on a lower copayment tier, but is being moved to or was moved to a higher copayment tier (tiering exception).*

☐ I want to be reimbursed for a covered prescription drug that I paid for out of pocket.

---

*NOTE: If you are asking for a formulary or tiering exception, your PRESCRIBING PHYSICIAN must provide a statement to support your request. You cannot ask for a tiering exception for a drug in the plan's Specialty Tier. In addition, you cannot obtain a brand name drug at the copayment that applies to generic drugs.

Additional information we should consider *(attach any supporting documents)*:

_____
_____
_____
_____

If you, or your prescribing physician, believe that waiting for a standard decision (which will be provided within 72 hours) could seriously harm your life or health or ability to regain maximum function, you can ask for an expedited (fast) decision. If your prescribing physician asks for a faster decision for you, or supports you in asking for one by stating (in writing or in a telephone call to us) that he or she agrees that waiting 72 hours could seriously harm your life or health or ability to regain maximum function, we will give you a decision within 24 hours. If you do not obtain your physician's support, we will decide if your health condition requires a fast decision.

☐ I need an expedited coverage determination (attach physician's supporting statement, if applicable)

_____   _____
Beneficiary/Requestor's Signature   Date

Send this request to your Medicare drug plan. Note that your Medicare drug plan may require additional information. See your plan benefit materials for more information.

Information on this form is protected health information and subject to all privacy and security regulations under HIPAA.

Figure 7–1   (continued)—page 3

- Drugs that a manufacturer requires that associated tests or monitoring services be purchased exclusively from the manufacturer or its designee as a condition of sale
- Barbiturates
- Benzodiazepines

Part D plan sponsors may by choice include these drugs as a supplemental drug covered under the plan they sponsor. This is under only "special circumstances."

Formularies Used to Lower Costs

Prescription drug plans are allowed to utilize drug formularies under Medicare Part D. Formularies are the central part of the PDPs efforts to reduce costs in the program by controlling how many drugs are eligible to be used. There is a requirement to have some drugs from every class of drugs, but not to cover all the drugs that are in a class.

An example may make this situation clearer. Let's say there are 40 drugs that can be used to treat high blood pressure. In order to reduce costs to you, the PDP may decide to cover only 6 of these 40 drugs. Also, with the 6 drugs that are chosen for the class, there may be 5 different dosage forms for each drug. The PDP may choose to cover only selected numbers of these differing dosage forms. So, it is really important for you to examine closely the plan that you choose and to select one that allows you to continue with the medications you currently take.

An example from another product line may help clarify the formulary concept. Think of the case when you buy bread from a grocery store or supermarket. Some stores have many different brands of bread and numerous sized loaves for each brand of bread stocked in the store. Other stores may only stock certain brands of bread and a more limited selection of sizes of the brand name breads. The hope for you is that you can find the type of bread that you like from the selection presented, even though not all brands of bread are stocked. This same concept is behind the formularies in Medicare Part D drug programs. With a more limited selection within a drug class, the plan can hopefully negotiate a better price with the manufacturer, and pass savings along to you when you obtain your prescriptions. CMS requires each Part D plan to provide some, not all, drugs within a class of drugs to treat a disease. Your specific drug may not be included, so it is important to check thoroughly before you sign up for a plan. If the drug is not covered under the plan, you have the right (regardless of which plan you are enrolled in) to petition to have the drug covered by your plan.

Specific Other Formulary Issues

There are several things that may be required before you can be prescribed certain drugs within the Part D program. These need to be explained. They include:

- Step therapy
- Prior authorization
- Preferred drug lists
- Tiered co-payments
- Pharmacy networks
- Dispensing limits

Step therapy. Step therapy occurs when you have to try one medication and see if it works or not for your condition before trying a more expensive drug. In the case of blood pressure medications, there may be an older drug that must be tried before a newer drug can be prescribed. The goal of step therapies is to try one medication on a short term basis (usually a less expensive drug) before prescribing you a newer and more expensive drug. You should look at the drug plan that you choose carefully. Examine what the policy is regarding step therapy and associated requirements.

Prior authorization. Prior authorization is a requirement that the drug plan must approve the use of a particular drug before your doctor can prescribe it for you. The drug in question may be an expensive drug. There may also be less expensive alternatives that may be equally effective. The

Not all formularies are the same. Some drug plans may cover more drugs than others do.

The Formularies In This Program, and How They Work

plan that you choose will spell out what the policy is regarding prior authorization.

Preferred drug lists. Prescription drug plans may have listings of drugs that are referred to as "preferred drug lists." For drugs on this list, your co-payment if you are required to pay a co-payment may be less than the amount that you have to pay if a drug is not on this listing. If your doctor disagrees with this, you can petition to have the drug paid for with the same co-payment as the preferred drugs. So, you may have to pay a varying amount of a co-payment depending upon whether the drug is classified as "preferred" or "non-preferred" by the drug plan. If you qualify for extra help under Medicare Part D, this varying co-payment may not affect you at all.

Tiered co-payments. "Tiered co-payments" refer to different amounts that you would pay as a co-payment. The way this works is if you are taking a generic medication, your co-payment would be the lowest. Next, you may pay a higher co-payment for a "preferred drug." See above definition. Finally, if you use a brand name drug, you will pay a higher co-payment over the previous two categories (generic, then preferred drug). Finally, if you are prescribed a drug for a condition for which it has not been approved, you may be required to pay the entire amount for the prescription. Doctors may prescribe a drug for any reason, even if the drug has not been approved to treat the condition that you have. This is called "off label" prescribing. You should know if you are taking any such drugs, so ask your doctor. And if you are taking "off label" drugs, can you perhaps be prescribed another drug for which you can pay a co-payment that is in one of the other lower priced co-payment tiers.

Pharmacy networks. Some of the Medicare Part D drug plans, or Medicare Advantage plans, may limit the places where you can obtain your new and refill prescriptions. I would advise you to check with your pharmacist before you sign up for a plan to see whether or not you can continue to use a particular pharmacy for your prescription needs. Having said this, many pharmacies will participate in all of the drug plans available to them. Many of the national chain community pharmacies or supermarket pharmacies are in this category. They provide national coverage for your needs.

Dispensing limits.   Your prescription drug plan may limit the amount of a prescription that you obtain. You may be restricted to a 30 day supply of the medications, even if you take the drug every day and will do so for a long period of time. There might be a mail order option with your drug plan, and if so, you may be able to obtain larger amounts of the prescription if you use this mail order option. This will vary from plan to plan. If this is an important issue for you, be sure to ask about this before you sign up for a prescription drug plan.

Summary of Formulary Issues

To summarize the issues surrounding formularies, spend some time thinking about the following issues. Determine if the drugs that you currently take are covered under a plan you are considering. If the drug is not covered, you and your doctor can petition to have the drug covered, and have an answer within 24 hours. Your doctor will fill out most of the form, make sure you know where or to whom at the drug plan to send the form. It is not sent to CMS, it is sent to the prescription drug plan, so find out if your doctor can fax the form for a speedier reply.

If you find during the course of your first year in a plan, that the plan is changing the formulary, and some of your drugs may no longer be covered under Medicare Part D, please know that during enrollment each year, you are entitled to change plans. You are not "stuck" with a plan that does not meet your needs.

Understand the concept of the "step therapy" process. Chances are you may have already been prescribed one of

$-Generic drugs
$$-Preferred drugs
$$$-Brand name drugs
$$$$-Off-label drugs

these "step therapies" and that is why you take the current drugs that you take! If this is the case, your doctor can contact the prescription drug plan, and let them know this has already been tried. You should *not* have to go through this again. It may be that the other therapy just did not work for you, or that you may have experienced a side effect that prohibits you from going through the process again.

Understand as much as you can about the policies of the prescription drug plan that deal with "prior approval" medications. Here once more, you may have already gone through this process before. Your doctor can help with the "prior approval" forms and take care of this along with your help. If you or your doctor feel strongly about a particular drug being right for you, be firm and assertive, and go through the channels set up to petition for coverage. Please consider that some of the drugs that you might be taking are not covered under Medicare Part D, and petitioning for having them approved will not work. Please refer to the listing of drug classes not eligible for coverage at the very front of this chapter.

Your drug plan may have preferred drug listing. If so, know what your rights are and realize that you may pay a higher amount for drugs that you take that are not on the preferred list. The "tiered co-payment" process means that you pay more for off label drugs than you would for brand name drugs which will be more expensive than preferred drugs which may be more expensive than generic prescriptions. You may not have the option to use a generic drug, but if you do you will pay less for the generic drug than you will for these other options.

Finally, check to make sure that you can use the pharmacy that you normally use for your prescription needs. Not all pharmacies are participating in all the various prescription drug plans. Make sure that you have a pharmacy that you can use for your prescriptions!

References

1. Medicare Part D §423.153(d).

CHAPTER 8

The Medication Management Programs and How To Use Them To Your Advantage

Medication Therapy Management Services

The Goal Is to Help with Your Medicine Taking

Besides proving savings for prescription medications, there is another important service that Medicare will pay for. There is a part of Medicare Part D termed medication therapy management services (MTMS) that will help you with taking your medications. The CMS legislation specifically noted that prescription drug plans must provide the following in an established MTMS program:[1]

- Ensuring optimum outcomes for beneficiaries who need services over and above regular services
- Reducing risks for adverse drug events
- Provides a means to provide fees for pharmacist and others to provide such services
- Pharmacists and other qualified providers to provide such services

- Provide opportunities for different services in hospital, nursing home, or outpatient areas
- Providing a program that is coordinated with chronic care improvement programs (CCIPs)

Who Is Eligible

You may be eligible for such services if you have several chronic diseases, such as high blood pressure, diabetes, and heart failure as a few examples. You also must be taking several drugs at the same time. Finally, you will need to have drug bills that are around $4,000 per year. If you meet these three qualifications, you may be eligible for extra help in taking your medication, including extra education, special compliance packaging, or other enhanced types of services.

It is important to find out before you sign up for a plan if you might be eligible for these services. Your doctor and pharmacist can help you if you need help. Also, check to see what services are provided with the specific plan that you might have in mind.

Your Rights

You have rights in these types of programs. Once you enroll, you are eligible to remain in the program throughout the balance of the year you are enrolled. This is the case even if you are able to increase your compliance, reduce the number of drugs you take, or have some other success as a result of being in these programs (see Table 8–1).

Table 8–1   Medication Therapy Management Services:
• Are for patients who take several drugs
• Have diseases that are chronic (long-term, or lifetime)
• Pay a lot for drugs each year
• Are meant to help you get the most from your medications that you possibly can
• Help to reduce your risk of experiencing an adverse drug reaction
• Will help you be more compliant with your drug

An Example of How It Would Work

Let's work through an example to see how this might work for you. Assume that you will spend $4,200 this year on your medications. You have had several infections and have taken several courses of really expensive medications. You have several chronic health conditions that require you to take numerous medications. For this example assume that you have to take:

- One tablet a day for your heart failure
- Two tablets a day to help your kidneys work
- One tablet a day to thin your blood
- One capsule a day to regulate your heart
- One tablet a day for your blood sugar
- One insulin shot after breakfast for your blood sugar
- Three tablets a day for high blood pressure
- Three puffs a day from an inhaler to help you breathe

For most days it is really hard for you to remember what you have taken and when you took your drugs. Who would not have trouble remembering all of this information? In addition, you have to check your blood sugar with a glucose monitor after every meal. You also have a salt free diet that you are to follow. You are 15 pounds overweight and you smoke a pack and a half of cigarettes a day.

This is an *exaggerated* example, but I would like to use it to speak about what is available to you for treatment. It is important to note that you will not have to pay extra for these services intended to help you. You are not to be charged an extra fee for the extra things that are done to help you. The prescription drug plan will pay the providers of the service; it may be a pharmacist or another professional who provides these services to you. If you are prescribed nicotine patches to help you stop smoking, they will be prescribed for you. Your prescription drug plan will provide this prescription to you through your pharmacy in the same manner that you receive the other drugs you take. You might be required to pay a co-payment or a small fee for the prescription. In any case, the cost to you will be less than you otherwise might have to pay.

How This Service Might Work for You

Initially you will be interviewed and a general plan developed to help you take your medicines and achieve the best results with the drugs you take. You may be provided a listing of your drugs and when you should take them, and there might be a place for you to put a check mark or other means to let you know that you have taken the drugs as you should.

Your medications may be packaged in a specialized manner to allow you to see what you need to take, and when you need to take doses. The package you see below is an example of what this might look like. This particular company is Medicine-on-Time® and this particular compliance packaging is an example of what your medicines might be dispensed in (Figures 8–1 to 8–3).

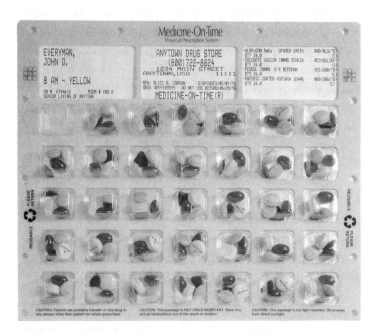

Figure 8–1   Example of Medicine-on-Time® Compliance Packaging
Source: Photographs provided with the approval of Medicine-on-Time®

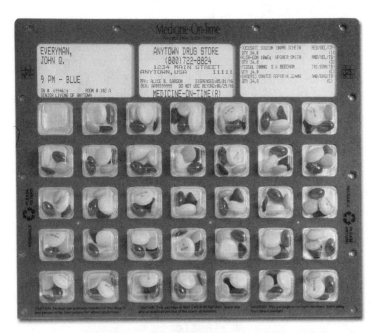

Figure 8–2   Example of a Medicine-on-Time® Color-coded Card for Time-of-day Administration

Source: Photographs provided with the approval of Medicine-on-Time®

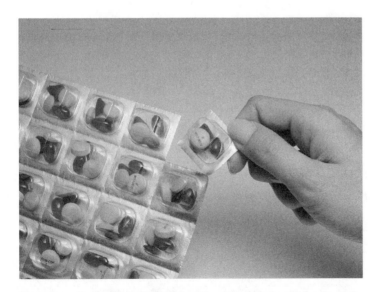

Figure 8–3   Example of a Medicine-on-Time® Package Containing Several Drugs To Be Taken Together at the Same Time

Source: Photographs provided with the approval of Medicine-on-Time®

105

By combining the products to be taken at the same time, compliance is accomplished. You will always be able to tell if you have taken the drugs that you should have. This system eliminates the need to have multiple bottles for all your medications. Your medications in this system are provided in this easy to see and easy to administer packaging. The individual packets for administration at specific times are all labeled with the names of the drug. These packages are also heat, light, and moisture resistant. The packages are also very easy to open and take the drugs from the cup that is covered by the label that seals the small packets (Figures 8–4 to 8–7).

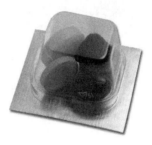

Figure 8–4   A Medicine-on-Time® Dose Container With Several Doses Taken at the Same Time
Source: Photographs provided with the approval of Medicine-on-Time®

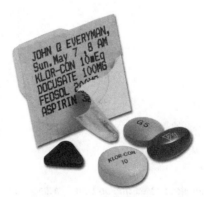

Figure 8–5   This Is What the Small Medicine-on-Time® Packets Look Like
Source: Photographs provided with the approval of Medicine-on-Time®

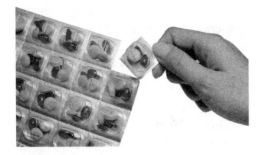

Figure 8–6   Example of a Medicine-on-Time® Prescription Package
Source: Photographs provided with the approval of Medicine-on-Time®

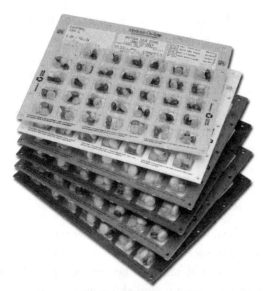

Figure 8–7   Example of Differing Administration Times Color Coded in the A Medicine-on-Time® System
Source: Photographs provided with the approval of Medicine-on-Time®

Specialized Contacts to You By Phone or in Person

You may also be asked to either call in every day, or be available for someone to call you to see how you are taking your medicine. This specialized contact is intended to help you with questions you might have, or to provide individualized help to you with taking your drugs. You might also have other services provided that are educational in nature and will allow

107

you to see better ways to follow the drug regimens that you have been prescribed. You might be asked to have appointments made for you to see the person providing the services to you. It will all depend on the situation that is specific to your needs. When these services are provided to you, your doctor will be kept up to date on what specifically has been provided to you, and what the actual benefits have been. In this way all providing care to you are kept informed as these services are provided to you.

Reducing the Number of Drugs That You Take

It might also be the case that you may not need to take as many drugs as you do now, and the total amount of drugs that you are required to take may change. There might be certain times of the day that you will take a certain number of drugs. This whole process is designed to simplify very complex regimens into something that you can manage more easily. Please see Appendix E 'Websites for more information about drugs' for a listing of websites with more information about drugs.

Use These Services If You Can

If you are offered these additional no cost services, I encourage you to use them to your advantage. Again, let me repeat the point that you should not be charged extra for any of these services. They are provided to you as a service paid for by the prescription drug plan. If someone does try to charge you for these services they are being deceitful and you should report them to the CMS.

References

1. Medicare Part D §423.153(d).

CHAPTER 9

Coverage for Preventive Services in the Medicare Program

Disease Prevention and Health Promotion

Disease Prevention

Medicare realizes how important your health is, and has implemented payment for services to help you stay in the best state of health that you can possibly achieve.[1-4] Prevention of disease is a very important way for you to stay healthy. Proper diet, exercise, keeping your weight down, and not smoking (or quitting smoking) are all things that you can do to prevent health problems. There are also some doctor initiated things that you should consider. One way to make the most of preventive services is to work with your doctor to have health "screenings" done. Screenings are tests that are done to check to see if you have a disease, or to monitor certain aspects of a disease if you have one. These prevention services may also identify risk factors for diseases that are present. Preventive services also include obtaining vaccinations (shots) to prevent a disease or condition from occurring. There are some services available to both men and women. There are also gender specific screenings for males or females.

Seniors Not Aware of Services Available

A major reason for this change in the Medicare program toward more preventive services lies in the fact that so many seniors are unaware of the services that are available. I am not blaming seniors; in most cases people do not know what is available to them. This is not their fault. CMS has noted that many services are so much underutilized. Consider the following rates of use for certain preventive services:

- 64% of women do not have Pap tests and pelvic exams to screen for cervical and uterine cancer
- 46% of men do not have regular PSA (prostate specific antigen) tests to detect prostate cancer
- 45% of women do not have regular mammograms
- 35% of Medicare recipients have not had a vaccination for pneumonia
- 32% do not obtain a flu shot yearly
- 17% have not had cholesterol tests done to screen for heart disease.

Medicare Will Pay for Screening Tests and Other Services for Beneficiaries

Medicare will pay for screening tests and other services for beneficiaries. For some of these services, you will have to meet the standard Medicare deductible. You will then pay 20% of the amount after the yearly deductible is paid. You can check the Medicare website www.cms.gov for more information. Also, there is a feature on the Medicare website: my.medicare.gov. According to information available on the site, this site is secure and online allowing you to access your Medicare information. You will have to register to use this service by entering your Medicare number and provide several other bits of information. You will need to supply:

- Medicare Number
- Last Name

- Date of Birth
- Gender
- Zip Code
- Shared Secret Question (you will pick from a list)
- Shared Answer
- e-mail address (optional only)
- Your relationship to beneficiary (if you are not the one filling out the form)
- Your Name (if you are someone other than self)

My.medicare.gov

Once you mail the form to CMS, you will be sent a letter within two weeks providing you with a password that you can use to access the services available. You can then access some of your personal data on the site my.medicare.gov. You will not be able to access your prescription information, but you will be able to:

- View claim status (but not Part D claims for prescriptions)
- Order a duplicate Medicare Summary Notice (MSN) or replacement Medicare card
- View eligibility, entitlement and preventive services information
- View enrollment information including prescription drug plans
- View or modify your drug list and pharmacy information
- View address of record with Medicare and Part B deductible status
- Access online forms, publications and messages sent to you by CMS.

I encourage you to use this site and look at your information often.

Health Promotion Screenings and Tests

Physical Examination (Women and Men). Newly covered preventive services include a one-time "Welcome to Medicare" physical exam. This will include an examination by your doctor, shots that you might need to have, and blood level screenings. There is a charge to you for this exam. You are eligible for this benefit within the first six months after you enroll in Medicare Part B. There is a time limit in that only those who began Medicare Part B coverage on or after January 1, 2005 are eligible. You will be charged a 20% co-payment of the approved amount after you have reached your Medicare Part B deductible.

Cardiovascular tests (Women and Men). You can also have several heart screening tests run. These tests are for your cholesterol, lipid, and triglyceride levels. These tests are done at no cost to you. If elevated, each of these has a potential damaging effect on your heart. Again, this is only for those enrolling in Medicare Part B after January 1, 2005.

Diabetes screening, supplies, and self-management training (Women and Men). Medicare covers diabetes screenings for all people with Medicare who are at risk for diabetes. You can have blood sugar levels drawn by your doctor at no cost to you. Again, this is only for those enrolling in Medicare Part B after January 1, 2005. If you have diabetes (high blood sugar) you can obtain blood sugar monitors (glucose monitors), test strips, and lancets at a 20% co-payment rate. If you have Medicare Part D and you use insulin shots, the insulin is covered under the prescription drug plan. If you are at risk for complications from diabetes, your doctor can request that you be provided diabetes self-management training. You will need to pay a 20% co-payment for these items and services.

For people with diabetes, Medicare covers certain services and supplies to treat diabetes and help prevent its complications. In most cases, your doctor must write an order or referral for you to get these services. These services include diabetes self-management training and medical nutrition therapy, under certain conditions.

Medicare will also pay for diabetic supplies, including blood sugar monitors, lancets, and testing strips, whether or not you are insulin dependent. Insulin and supplies used to inject it are covered under Medicare's prescription drug coverage.

For people with diabetes, Medicare also covers hemoglobin A1c tests (a blood test to measure how well your blood sugar has been controlled over the past 3 months), and special eye exams. This hemoglobin A1c test is a way for your doctor to follow your progress over a period of time and gives a better picture of long-term control of your diabetes.

Medicare also covers insulin pumps, special foot care, and therapeutic shoes for people with diabetes who need them.

So, what do you have to pay? In the Original Medicare Plan, you pay 20% of the Medicare-approved amount after the annual Part B deductible for diabetes training, a monitor, lancets, and test strips, as well as medical nutrition therapy. For more information, get a free copy of *Medicare Coverage of Diabetes Supplies & Services* (CMS Pub. No. 11022) at www.medicare.gov on the web. Select "Publications."

Breast Cancer Screenings—Mammograms (Women). Breast cancer is the second leading cause of deaths for women in the United States. Early detection by use of mammograms can help to identify breast cancer at early stages. Treatment has a better success rate if the cancer is diagnosed early. Once every year, women are eligible for a mammogram if they have Medicare and are older than 40 years of age. You will have to pay a 20% co-payment for the yearly mammogram. You are at a higher risk for breast cancer occurrence if you have never had a child, had your first child after 30 years

Coverage for Preventive Services in the Medicare Program

of age, have had breast cancer before, and/or if you have a history of breast cancer in your family history.

Bone Mass Measurement. You *will have to pay a 20% co-payment after the yearly Part B deductible.* This screening can be done once every two years unless it is medically necessary to do this more often.

Risk factors for osteoporosis include:

- 50 years of age or older
- Female
- Family history of broken bones
- White or Asian
- Small-bone frame individuals
- Have a low body weight
- Smoke
- Excessive diet
- A low calcium diet

Glaucoma tests. *You will have to pay a 20% co-payment after the yearly Part B deductible.* This screening can be done once every year. This test analyzes the blood pressure in your eyes. Regular eye exams are the best way to head off potential problems with glaucoma.

Risk factors for glaucoma include:

- Diabetes
- Family history of glaucoma
- African-American descent
- Being 50 years of age or older

Cervical and Vaginal Cancer Screening (Women). Women can have these important screening procedures done. Medicare will pay for Pap tests and pelvic examinations to check for cancer of the cervix or vagina. These tests can be done every two years. Medicare will pay the complete costs of the Pap lab test. It will cost a 20% co-payment for the examinations and collection of the Pap test.

Having an infection called human papillomavirus (HPV) is the most common cause of cervical cancer. Not all women with HPV infections develop cervical cancer. A regular Pap test can help to identify the cancer at an early stage. The Pap test can detect pre-cancerous and cancerous cells on your cervix. Other risk factors for cervical and vaginal cancer also include the following:

- Giving birth to many children
- Having many sexual partners
- Having first sexual intercourse at a young age
- Smoking cigarettes
- Oral contraceptive use ("the Pill")
- Having a weakened immune system

Symptoms include:

- Vaginal bleeding
- Unusual vaginal discharge
- Pelvic pain
- Pain during sexual intercourse

Colorectal cancer screening (Women and Men). Medicare pays for screenings done to detect colorectal cancer. The rates of colorectal cancer increase after we reach the age of 50 years. As with other cancers, early detection is the key to treatment success. The purpose of screening is to identify what are called polyps. These are growths in the colon that are termed pre-cancerous. They can be clipped out before they cause full blown cancer of the colon.

There are several tests that are covered. I will list each one, and then list the co-payment that is required to be paid by you. These are available for persons with Medicare and are over the age of 50 years of age.

Fecal Occult Blood Test. This annual test is no cost to you.

Flexible Sigmoidoscopy. There is a charge of *20% of the approved Medicare rate after the yearly deductible.* If done in a hospital outpatient department, *the fee is 25% of the Medicare-approved rate.* This can be tested once every 4 years

Screening Colonoscopy. There is a charge *20% of the approved Medicare rate after the yearly deductible.* If done in a hospital outpatient department, *the fee is 25% of the Medicare-approved rate.* This can be tested once every two years if you happen to be at high risk. If you are not at a high risk, once every ten years you can have this test. You can not have coverage if you have had a flexible sigmoidoscopy within four years and are not at high risk for colorectal cancer.

Barium Enema. *You will have to pay a 20% co-payment after the yearly Part B deductible.* Your doctor may choose to perform this rather than the flexible sigmoidoscopy or screening colonoscopy. This test is covered every two years if you are at a high risk for colorectal cancer, and every four years if you are not at a high risk for colorectal cancer.

Risk factors for colorectal cancer include:

- Family history of either polyps or colon cancer
- Inflammatory bowel disease, such as ulcerative colitis or Crohn's disease
- A diet that is high in fat (such as meats)
- Physical inactivity
- Obesity
- Smoking
- Alcohol intake (colorectal cancer has been linked to the heavy use of alcohol)

Prostate cancer screening (Men). Prostate cancer can be detected early by a test examining the amount of prostate specific antigen (PSA) in the blood. Another test is when your doctor performs a digital rectal examination. These two tests and associated fees are listed below. There are several tests that are covered. I will list each one, and then list the co-payment that is required to be paid by you.

Digital Rectal Examination. *You will have to pay a 20% co-payment after the yearly Part B deductible.* This test is covered once every year.

Prostate Specific Antigen (PSA) test. There is no cost to you. This test is once every year.

Risk factors for prostate cancer are highest for African Americans, followed by Whites, Hispanics, Asians, Pacific Islanders, and followed by Native Americans.

Other risk factors include:

- A diet high in red meat or high fats
- Lack of exercise
- Smoking
- High alcohol consumption
- Having had a vasectomy when younger than age 35 years (this is still a controversial and debated linkage)

Various shots (Vaccinations) for Flu, Pneumococcal Pneumonia, Hepatitis B. These shots are important for seniors to have to protect against serious infections. All seniors should obtain a flu shot every year, and for most people a pneumonia vaccination one time. There are several shots that are covered. I will list each one, and then list the co-payment that is required to be paid by you.

Flu shot. *There is no cost to you.* You should obtain this every year, either in the fall or winter.

Pneumococcal shot. *There is no cost to you.* Most seniors only need this vaccination one time in their life.

Hepatitis B shots. *You will have to pay a 20% co-payment after the yearly Part B deductible.* This vaccination will require you to have three shots. This vaccination is for individuals with a medium to high risk of contracting Hepatitis B. This series of three shots are administered once in your life. Risk factors for Hepatitis B include end stage renal disease, hemophilia, lowered resistance to infections.

Smoking Cessation Counseling

Smoking kills plain and simple. Cigarette smoking kills almost 500,000 persons per year. This number includes active smokers who smoke themselves, and passive smokers who are those who inhale other's smoke (second-hand smoke). Regardless of how old you are, quitting smoking will benefit you and those around you. Quitting smoking has significant benefits for you, even if you are an older adult and have smoked for years. Please think about quitting smoking. It is the hardest thing in the world to quit, because nicotine in cigarettes is a very addictive drug. But if you quit you will help yourself, serve as a role model for others, and realize you have done something really great!

Smoking causes numerous health problems. Smoking causes many health problems including:

- Allergies
- Cataracts
- Depression
- Gastrointestinal disease
  - Ulcers
  - Stomach cancer
- Heart disease
  - Heart attacks
  - Angina pectoris
  - Congestive heart failure
  - High blood pressure (hypertension)

- Alzheimer's disease
- Periodontal disease (dental diseases: gums, teeth, tongue)
- Periodontal disease
- Peripheral vascular disease
  - Blood clots
  - Deep vein thrombosis
- Strokes
- Worsening of diabetes
- Breathing problems
  - Emphysema
  - Asthma
  - Bronchitis
  - Frequent respiratory tract infections
- Cancer
  - Virtually every form of cancer can be caused by smoking. Prominent cancers with a smoking linkage include:
    - ☐ Breast
    - ☐ Esophageal
    - ☐ Larynx
    - ☐ Lung
    - ☐ Kidney
    - ☐ Mouth
    - ☐ Leukemia
    - ☐ Lymphoma
    - ☐ Pancreatic
    - ☐ Prostate
    - ☐ Stomach
    - ☐ Skin
    - ☐ Testicular
    - ☐ Throat

Coverage of smoking cessation counseling. Smoking cessation counseling is covered for Medicare enrollees who have an illness that is caused or complicated by smoking. Also, those who take drugs affected by tobacco use have this benefit. Services offered include smoking cessation counseling (this can be provided as an outpatient or as an inpatient in a hospital). There are levels of intensity of the counseling that are also paid for. Smoking cessation drug therapies may also be paid for by Medicare.

Drugs do not work as well when you smoke. There are many drug therapies that are negatively impacted by smoking. Some of these therapies include:

- Blood pressure medications do not work as well if you smoke
- Medications taken for diabetes do not work as well if you smoke
  - Insulin
  - Oral insulin drugs (oral hypoglycemic drugs)
- Drugs taken for breathing problems
  - Asthma drugs
  - Emphysema drugs
- Antibiotics
  - Drugs taken to treat infections
- Pain relief medications
  - All types of pain relievers:
    - ☐ Minor analgesics
    - ☐ Prescription strength pain relievers
    - ☐ Anti-arthritic drugs
    - ☐ Narcotic analgesics, those that contain drugs such as codeine, hydrocodone, etc.

As this list above indicates, many drugs just do not work as well if you smoke. Ask your doctor to help you quit smoking for many reasons. If your drugs are treating a chronic condition (cardiovascular or heart disease), seek help with smoking cessation counseling. If you have frequent lung infections, respiratory tract infections, or other breathing related infections, please ask your doctor to help you get counseling to quit smoking.

What Specific Services Are Provided to Help You Stop Smoking?

I will list each of the covered smoking cessation services, and then list the co-payment that is required to be paid by you.

Counseling. *You will have to pay a 20% co-payment after the yearly Part B deductible.* You can receive up to eight counseling sessions per year. It may take multiple sessions for you to be able to quit smoking. Keep at it, and do not become discouraged. If you know someone who has Medicare coverage and smokes, this is a great motivator for you to present to them to allow them to see that there are tools for them to help them quit smoking.

Medicare Part D coverage for smoking cessation drug therapies. Medicare Part D will pay for nicotine patches. These are the patches that you apply once a day to help people quit smoking. These are the nicotine patches. Even if you have used these patches in the past, and no longer do, you may benefit by using this tool to help you quit smoking.

New Health Promotion and Disease Prevention Services for 2007

In 2007, Medicare will add:

- Ultrasound screening coverage for abdominal aortic aneurysms (based on a referral from the "Welcome to Medicare" physical exam) with no deductible. The aorta is the largest artery in your body, and it carries blood away from your heart. When it reaches your abdomen, it is called the abdominal aorta. The abdominal aorta supplies blood to the lower part of the body. Just below the abdomen, the aorta splits into two branches that carry blood into each leg. When a weak area of the abdominal aorta expands or bulges, it is called an abdominal aortic aneurysm.

- No deductible for colorectal cancer screening in the Original Medicare Plan

Use These Services to Help Yourself to Better Health

This chapter has presented a summary of preventive services available to you as a person with Medicare. Some of the above coverage for preventive services is new to the Medicare Program. Through these prevention activities, the hope is that you can remain in the best possible health for as long as you possibly can!

References

1. Centers for Disease Control and Prevention, website accessed, August 10, 2006 at: http://www.cancer.gov/cancertopics/pdq/treatment/cervical/#Keypoint6
2. *Guide to Medicare's Preventive Services*, CMS-10110, Centers for Medicare and Medicaid Services; August, 2004.
   My.Medicare.gov, accessed August 10, 2006.
3. *Staying Healthy Medicare's Preventive Services*, CMS-11100, Centers for Medicare and Medicaid Services; December, 2004.
4. *Medicare Coverage of Diabetes Supplies & Services* (CMS Pub. No. 11022) at www.medicare.gov on the internet. Centers for Medicare and Medicaid Service, September, 2004.

CHAPTER 10

Getting Your Drugs and Drug Taking in Order

Tips to Improve Your Drug Taking

I have noted several times some things for you to think about before you begin the process of signing up for Medicare Part D. These items are related to the drugs that you take, some new aspects of the Medicare Part D program, and some issues on how to change the plan you sign up for. These all are intended to help you with the next steps that you take to get the most out of this benefit.

I want to initially begin here by covering some things that you should think about with regard to the drugs that you currently take. I would encourage you seek to limit the number of drugs that you take. Granted this is not always possible. There may be generic drugs that you can take as well that might save you money. Let me start by going over some things for you to think about when you look at the drugs you take and how you take them.

Take As Few Drugs As Possible

It is always a good practice to take as few drugs as possible. Some physicians who specialize in treating seniors, gerontologists, recommend reducing the number of drugs you take as much as can be done. Some suggest, as the following diagram indicates, that after a person takes eight drugs total per day, one drug needs to be stopped before another can be prescribed. Now this is just a rule of thumb. You may need to take this many drugs for very good reasons. This is something that you and your doctor need to discuss and come to an agreement. You should always feel free to ask your doctor to clarify something or to consider something that you suggest. The more that you can participate in the decisions made about your health, the better your health will be and the chances are that your drugs will work better too. Please see Figure 10–1 for a graphic depiction of what you might do if you take eight or more medicines.

Routine Check-ups

You tune your car and your appliances. You also can fine tune your medicine taking habits. In other words, have your medicines checked regularly by your doctors and pharmacists. Once every 6–12 months, have your doctors and pharmacists review all the drugs that you take. Your pharmacist will know the drugs that you take from the pharmacy where they work,

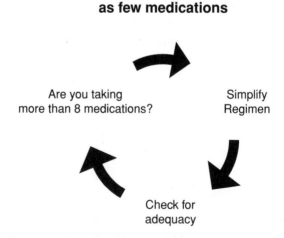

When at all possible – take as few medications

Are you taking more than 8 medications?

Simplify Regimen

Check for adequacy

Figure 10–1   Taking As Few Medications As Possible

but not from elsewhere. So, it is vital that you let your care-givers know what other prescription drugs you are taking from all sources. Your doctors will know what drugs are prescribed by them, but not from other doctors or dentists that you see for care. Also, let all your caregivers know the over-the-counter drugs you take. These are the drugs that you can buy without a prescription. You may also be taking herbal remedies, vitamin supplements, or tonics. Always let your pharmacists and doctors know that you are taking these too. Consumer Reports[1] *OnHealth* suggests that you double-check for needless drugs if you take five or more drugs, have more than three health problems, have several doctors write prescriptions for you, have not reviewed all your drugs and supplements taken with your primary care doctor in the past six months, have been hospitalized recently, and/or take a drug for a month or more that can lead to addiction. These drugs might include narcotic pain relievers, drugs to help you sleep at night, and cough syrups that contain codeine or related compounds. Here again, your pharmacist can help you with these items as well.

What Is Patient Compliance?

Patient compliance with medications and regimens is a part of the process of drug use by patients. The prescribed drugs that patients take can be a small part of total drug use by patients. Other drugs taken may include over-the-counter (OTC) drugs, herbal supplements, vitamins, nutritional supplements, and perhaps drugs borrowed from other friends, family members, or perfect strangers. Taking drugs on a regularly scheduled basis is a difficult task. As a matter of fact, 50% of us are not compliant at any one point in time with the drugs that we take. Many things occur in our lives that divert our attention readily to other pressing matters. It is so easy to be critical of ourselves or others that have trouble with taking medications as scheduled. But take it easy on yourself! Many times the dosing and frequency of administration of drugs can be confusing and bewildering.

Various Forms of Patient Compliance

There are several forms of medication compliance behavior. These range from obtaining your medications after your doctor writes your prescriptions (initial compliance), to taking part of your drugs. The average rate of compliance is 50% across all medication types! You can also be completely compliant and take all of your medications as you should all the time. Also, you can take too much of your medicines and be hypercompliant (too much of a good thing!). See Figure 10–2 for a depiction of the interrelatedness of compliance behavior.

The importance of patient compliance being the best it can be. How well you take your medications as prescribed can affect much of your health. The more compliant you are with

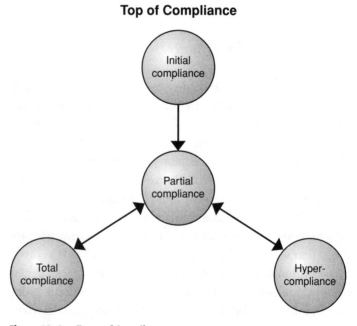

Figure 10–2   Types of Compliance

the drugs that you take the better your health will be. You may think that you already take too many drugs. But, if you do not take your drugs as prescribed you will have more health problems and be prescribed even more drugs. That is why with this drug benefit you have to really take the drugs prescribed for you in the best manner possible. The fewer drugs taken by you will also save you money by postponing the need to take other drugs. The more drugs that you take, the more money you spend. So controlling the drugs that you are taking now allows you to benefit in better health, lower costs for drugs, and avoiding other costs in the future. How you take your drugs is called patient compliance with medications and regimens. The prescribed drugs that you take can be a small part of your total drug use. Other drugs taken may include over-the-counter (OTC) drugs, herbal supplements, vitamins, nutritional supplements, and perhaps drugs borrowed from other friends, family members, or perfect strangers. For the most part and for most patients the fewer drugs that you take the better off you are. This does not mean taking less of the drugs prescribed for you. It means eliminating unnecessary future expenses for more drugs by taking your current drugs in the best manner that you can.

Difficulties seniors face with medication compliance. Sometimes it is difficult for seniors to be compliant with the drugs that you take. There are several reasons that include:

Social isolation. Many seniors live alone and it is hard when you are by yourself to remember when to take your medications. If you happen to live alone, think of a friend that can help you remember to take your drugs. They might be able to call you and you can do the same for them. Work with a "buddy" to help you remember. If you have a relative that lives close to you, or can call you, ask them to help you too.

Chronic disease. As we get older, there are more diseases that we have the potential to get. It is a blessing to have drugs that can prevent complications of disease if we take our medicines correctly. It can make you feel down when you have several conditions at the same time (for example, diabetes, high blood pressure, glaucoma, heart failure, etc.). I encourage you to be as well as you can be, even if you have numerous ailments. Taking your drugs as they have been prescribed is a good way to live your best in the state health you find yourself in.

Severity of disease.   When we have chronic diseases for a long period of time, the disease can become more severe over time. This is something that need not happen. There are things we can do to limit the outcomes of diseases that become worse and worse. Here again, being as compliant as you possibly can be will help you avoid complications of diseases down the road.

Multiple drug regimens.   The more ailments we have, often the more drugs are prescribed as a way to treat the disease. Taking more drugs can lead you to be less compliant than you could be. Here again, make it a part of your routine activities to take your drugs at the same time daily.

Complex drug regimens.   Finally, work with your pharmacist and doctors to help you simplify how you take your drugs. It may mean that you can be more compliant by combining your drugs that you take into segments that you can more easily remember. No one can be expected to be compliant 100% of the time. If you slip up and forget a dose, work harder to remember to take your drugs better the next day. Always ask for help and let others help you try to simplify your drug taking.

Advice on Medication Taking

Always discard your old or unused medications that have expired. Make it a part of your daily routine to take medications at a time that will be easy for you to remember. And as such, you will make it a habit of taking your drugs at the same time.

This might be in the morning, in the evening, or alongside another daily task. This could be taking your drugs after you brush your teeth. It might be in the morning around the time that you eat your breakfast. Or, it could be at night before you retire in the evening. If it is possible, write down somewhere that you have taken your drugs. This might be on a calendar, a diary, or a notebook.

Answers to Know About Your Medications

You should always know several important things about the medications that you take. You can ask your pharmacist for the answer to these questions. Also feel free to ask your doctor to explain answers to these questions:

- What is the name of the drug that I am taking?
- What does this drug look like? Are there different forms of this medication?
- What are the generic names for the drugs that I take?
- How should I take the medicine?
- How long should I continue to take the medication?
- What are some side effects that I need to watch out for?
- Will the drugs I take interact with each other, over-the-counter drugs that I take, or herbal supplements that I take?
- Is there a place I need to store this medication? Does it need to be refrigerated?
- Can I take this medication with food, vitamins, or alcoholic beverages?
- What happens if I miss a dose, when should I take the next one?
- When can I expect to see the results of taking this medication?

Please see Figure 10–3 (The connect the dots diagram).

Use this model to help yourself be as optimally compliant as you can. Always stop taking dangerous drugs that you no longer need to be taking. These might be strong pain pills

Never accept the directions: "Take as directed" or "As directed" on your prescriptions. Your physician and pharmacist need to explain in detail how you are to take any medicine. Keep asking until you receive proper directions.

Getting Your Drugs and Drug Taking in Order

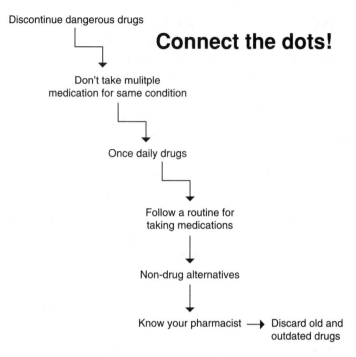

Figure 10–3   Connect the Dots with Your Medication

that you no long need to take. Do not take multiple drugs for the same condition unless asked to do so by your doctor. If at all possible take drugs that only require you to take one dose a day which will help you be more compliant. The less complex your medication taking is, the better chance you have to be compliant with your drug taking. If there is a non-drug alternative available to you, see if this can lead to taking less drugs. This might be a change in your diet, getting more exercise, or finding a way to have less stress in your life. I always feel it is best to know who your pharmacist is and to only shop at one pharmacy. Again, always discard your old drugs and certainly those drugs that are outdated need to be thrown away. You can always ask your pharmacist if your drugs are outdated, or have the pharmacist show you how you can tell if a drug is outdated and not usable any longer. Most prescriptions are now required to have an expiration date listed on the label itself. Ask you pharmacist to show you how to find this information easily on the label of your medicines.

Most prescriptions when dispensed have as a rule an expiration date that is listed as one year from the date of prescription filling. However, you may be dispensed a drug with a shorter amount of shelf life available, and if this is the case, the one year date is not correct. You will not know what the original expiration date is unless you ask the pharmacist. Just make sure that the drugs that you are receiving are in date and correctly marked. Some items such as ophthalmic (for use in the eye(s), or otic (for use in the ears) preparations have a shorter expiration date due to the way the items are used. For any ophthalmic preparation, I recommend that after 90 days you discard the remaining amount. You may not have to use the product for this length of time anyway. The tube or ointment may have an extended expiration date listed somewhere on the product itself. But, please note that once the sterile seal is broken as you open the product for the first time, this expiration date is invalid due to the sterility of the product now being less than listed. The expiration date put on these containers by the manufacturer assumes that the product is unopened and thus remains sterile. Once opened the sterility is lost.

See Appendix E for websites with more information about drugs.

Make sure that your doctor and pharmacist know all the medications that you are taking. These may be prescription, OTC, or herbal products. Regardless of type of medication, let your caregivers know all the drugs that you regularly take.

Summary

By getting your drug taking and your drug regimes in order, you can help yourself any number of ways. You can help to postpone additional health problems if you are as compliant as you can be with the number of drugs that you take. If you can help cut down the number of drugs that you take, this will help ease the complexity of the drug regimens that you have. It will also allow you the opportunity to simplify this part of your health care to a better extent.

Getting Your Drugs and Drug Taking in Order

Anything that we do to improve compliance will rarely be a 100% successful proposition. But most things that we do to become more compliant can improve health for all of us – me included! Your goal should be how to help you and yours become healthier by making the taking of medications easier and thus become more compliant with drug regimens. You cannot and should not be expected to do all of this on your own! Your doctors and pharmacists can help you devise the best medicine taking schedule that you deserve. Ask them to help you and please be persistent. I have said it before in this book, but you owe it to yourself. And, they owe it you too!

References

1. Taking more prescription drugs than you need? How to identify unnecessary, potentially harmful medications. *Consumer Reports On-Health*, Volume 18, Number 7, July 2006.

CHAPTER 11

Summary and Next Steps

So Where Do You Go from Here?

Where do you go from here with all of this? Let us now discuss some specific items about the Medicare Part D drug program and some new items effective for 2007. Costs will increase for the initial deductible amount, and for the amounts necessary to pay before catastrophic coverage begins. Please see the table below for information on how the amounts you will pay differ between 2006 and 2007. Keep in mind that costs will no doubt increase some each year hereafter as well. This is not unlike the premiums that you pay for regular Medicare coverage going up on a yearly basis.

Several Changes for 2007 and Beyond

Premium and deductible increases. As required by law, the parameters for the standard benefit are indexed to the increase in average total drug expenses of people with Medicare. The standard benefit is the minimum coverage plans must provide. (These amounts are subject to rounding.) Please see Table 11–1 for changes effective in 2007.

The limits will increase in 2007 as follows:

- Deductible from $250 in 2006 to $265 in 2007
- Initial coverage limit from $2,250 to $2,400 in 2007

Table 11–1   2007 Changes in Standard Benefit

Benefit Parameters	2006	2007
Deductible	$250	$265
Initial coverage limit	$2250	$2400
Out-of-pocket threshold	$3600	$3850
Total covered drugs at OOP threshold	$5100	$5451.25

LIS Copayments	2006	2007
Institutionalized	$0	$0
Up to or at 100% FPL	$1.00/$3.00	$1.00/$3.10
Other LIS	$2.00/$5.00	$2.15/$5.35

Abbreviations:
  Low income subsidy—LIS
  Out-of-pocket—OOP
  Federal poverty limit—FPL

Source: U.S. Centers for Medicare and Medicaid Services (CMS)

- Out-of-pocket threshold from $3,600 in 2006 to $3,850 in 2007
- Total out-of-pocket cost threshold from $5,100 in 2006 to $5,451.25 in 2007
- Minimum cost-sharing in catastrophic coverage from $2 in 2006 to $2.15 in 2007 for generic or preferred drugs and from $5.00 in 2006 to $5.35 in 2007 for all other drugs
- People with Medicare and full Medicaid benefits (full-benefit dual eligibles) who are institutionalized continue to pay nothing for Medicare-covered drugs.
- The maximum co-payments below the out-of-pocket threshold for full-benefit dual-eligible people with incomes up to 100% of the Federal poverty level are $1 for generic or preferred drugs (no change from 2006) and $3.10 (up from $3.00) for all other drugs in 2007.
- Other people eligible for the extra help (LIS = limited income subsidy) will pay $2.15 (up from $2.00) for generic/preferred drugs and $5.35 (up from $5.00) for all other drugs.

In addition, people who receive the partial subsidy will pay a $53.00 annual deductible (up from $50 in 2006) and will continue to pay cost-sharing of 15%.

Pilot programs for persons with chronic diseases. One of the aspects of the legislation that provides for Medicare Part D is another project to create a pilot project that supports co-ordinated care for people who are chronically ill.[1] Chronic conditions are one of the leading causes of illness, disability, and death among people with Medicare and lead to large and disproportionate costs for the Medicare program. These are chronic conditions such as high blood pressure, diabetes, heart failure, kidney disease, etc. This program providing what is called Medicare Health Support is designed to reduce health risks, to coordinate care, to help people with Medicare adhere to their physicians' plans of care, and to improve the quality of life for people living with chronic conditions such as heart failure or diabetes.

As of July, 2006 more than 115,000 people with Medicare have agreed to participate in the voluntary Medicare Health Support Programs. Medicare Health Support connects program participants with specially trained health care professionals who offer self-care guidance, answers to questions about health conditions or medications, coordination with locally available social services, as well as a 24-hour nurse telephone line. Participants remain in Original Medicare, and can keep their current physicians and providers. These are not Medicare Advantage or Part D Plans.

Medicare Health Support is designed as a two-phase initiative. Phase I is a pilot phase that will run for three years. Phase II is the expansion phase for Phase I programs or components that were successful in improving clinical quality outcomes, increasing participant satisfaction, and meeting Medicare spending targets for their assigned populations.

The project operates in a few select states, so take advantage of this program if there is one available to you and you qualify. This pilot is operating in the following eight areas:

- Oklahoma as of August 1, 2005 (Lifemasters)
- Washington, D.C., and Maryland as of August 1, 2005 (Healthways)
- Western Pennsylvania as of August 15, 2005 (Health Dialog)
- Mississippi as of August 22, 2005 (McKesson)
- Northwest Georgia as of September 12, 2005 (Cigna)
- Chicago, Illinois, as of September 1, 2005 (Aetna)
- Central Florida as of November 1, 2005 (Green Ribbon Health)
- Tennessee as of January 16, 2005 (XL Health)

Again these programs are available in a small number of states. Please think about signing up for one in your region if available.

Miscellaneous Medicare Provisions That Are New

There are several miscellaneous Medicare provisions that are new beginning in 2006 and 2007. These new segments deal with the following:

- Income-related increase in the Part B premium
- Health Savings Accounts
- Ombudsman program
- Medicaid eligibility

Income-related Increase in Part B Premium

Medicare has set new guidelines for increasing the Part B premium and deductible. Currently, that the Medicare Part B premium people have to pay is set at 25% of estimated program spending in a given year. A person's income has not been a basis for determining the premium.

However, beginning January 2007, the new Medicare Part B premium increase will be phased in for individuals with modified adjusted gross income of $80,000 or more and for couples filing a joint tax return with modified adjusted gross income of $160,000 or more. If the person meets the income threshold, the government's subsidy will be less than the current 75%. If the modified adjusted gross income for an individual is:

- Greater than $80,000 and not more than $100,000, the government subsidy is 65%
- Greater than $100,000 and not more than $150,000, the government subsidy is 50%
- Greater than $150,000 and not more than $200,000, the government subsidy is 35%
- Greater than $200,000, the government subsidy is 20%

The income ranges for joint returns are double that of individual returns.

For people whose income is above $80,000 (single) or $160,000 (married couple), Social Security will use the income reported two years ago on the income tax return to determine the Part B premium. For example, the income reported on a 2005 tax return will be used to determine the monthly Part B premium in 2007. Under certain circumstances people can ask that the income from a more recent tax year be used to determine the premium. At the end of 2006, Social Security will send a letter to people whose Part B premium will increase based on the level of their income, telling them about the change and what they can do if they disagree. For more information about premiums based on income, call Social Security at 1-800-772-1213. TTY users should call 1-800-325-0778.

Health Savings Accounts. To help with the rising costs of health care, Congress included provisions in the MMA legislation for establishing Health Savings Accounts (HSAs).[2] HSAs are tax-advantaged savings accounts that can be used to pay for medical expenses incurred by individuals and their families.

HSAs are available to anyone not entitled to Medicare who has a health insurance plan with a high deductible. HSA contributions and earnings are tax-free. The annual

137

deductible must be at least $1,050 for individual coverage and $2,100 for family coverage in 2006. The policy must also have a maximum limit on the annual deductible plus out-of-pocket medical expenses of $5,250 for individual coverage and $10,500 for family coverage in 2006. Out-of-pocket expenses include co-payments and other amounts, but do not include premiums. The policy may provide preventive care benefits without a deductible or with a deductible below the minimum annual deductible.

HSAs can be moved from one employer to another (they are portable), regardless of which job or employer a person may have. Contributions to an HSA made by a person's employer (including contributions made through a cafeteria plan) may be excluded from gross income. Like an individual retirement account (IRA), the individual owns the HSA, not the employer. If the person changes jobs, the HSA goes with the individual. Unused funds in an HSA may be carried over from one year to the next.

A HSA can be set up with a qualified HSA trustee such as a bank, an insurance company, or anyone approved by the IRS. Annual HSA contributions can be up to the amount of the plan's deductible but no more than $2,700 (self-only coverage) or $5,450 (family coverage) in 2006. These amounts are adjusted for the cost of living each year. Individuals age 55 and older can make extra contributions to their accounts.

The interest and earnings on the account are not taxable while in the HSA. Withdrawals are tax-free as long as the funds are used for qualified medical expenses, such as prescription and over-the-counter drugs, long-term care, or to purchase continued health care coverage under COBRA. Amounts withdrawn for other purposes will be taxable plus an additional 10% tax.

Once people are entitled to Medicare, they can no longer make HSA contributions. However, they can make tax-free medical expense withdrawals to pay co-payments required by Medicare or their Medicare Advantage plan, long-term care insurance premiums, and MA or Part D plan premiums if they are 65 or older. The law also allows health plans to offer Medicare Savings Accounts for people with Medicare.

Ombudsman

MMA authorized the appointment of a Medicare Beneficiary Ombudsman to ensure people with Medicare get the information and help they need to understand their Medicare options, including their rights and protections.[3] The Office of the Medicare Beneficiary Ombudsman will address processes for complaints and information request.

The Ombudsman works to ensure that existing Medicare information, counseling, and assistance resources work the way they should to help people with their complaints, appeals, grievances, or questions about Medicare. The Ombudsman also works with the State Health Insurance Assistance Programs to help people with Medicare regarding Medicare Advantage Plans and changes to those plans. The office submits an annual report to Congress and the Secretary of Health and Human Services describing activities and recommending changes to improve program administration.

The Ombudsman is not the initial contact for issues and complaints. The office will hold "open door forums" to provide information about the ombudsman program and what it can do for you as a Medicare enrollee. There are several points of contact for individual questions, complaints, and grievances, such as the toll-free Medicare helpline. Open Door Forums provide opportunities for people with Medicare, their caregivers, and advocates to publicly discuss with the Ombudsman their issues and concerns about Medicare systems and processes. People can sign up for the mailing list to participate in the Open Door Forums by clicking the link on the Ombudsman website.

MMA section 923 also required CMS to provide the toll-free telephone number 1-800-MEDICARE (1-800-633-4227) as the only number people need to call for Medicare information or assistance.

Proof of citizenship. The Deficit Reduction Act of 2005 requires states to obtain proof of United States citizenship and identity from people applying for, or re-enrolling in, Medicaid after July 1, 2006. United States citizenship or legal immigration status has always been required for Medicaid eligibility, but prior to July 2006, applicants could assert their status by checking a box on a form.

People receiving Medicare or supplement security income (SSI) benefits are exempt from the new requirement because they already had to establish their citizenship when they enrolled in those programs.

The list of acceptable documents is similar to the guidelines used by SSA to establish citizenship for determining SSI eligibility and issuing Social Security numbers. A single document (United States passport, Certificate of Naturalization, or Certificate of United States Citizenship) may be enough to establish both citizenship and identity. If a birth certificate or other document is used, the person will also need evidence of identity. Once citizenship has been proven, it need not be documented again unless later evidence raises a question. Current recipients should not lose benefits while they are undertaking a good-faith effort to provide documentation to the state.

Qualifying for extra help. People with Medicare who receive Medicaid benefits during the year, either full Medicaid benefits or partial (i.e., people in a Medicare Savings Program, who get help from Medicaid with their Medicare premiums/cost-sharing) automatically qualify for the extra help. CMS determines them to be eligible based on data received from the state. They qualify for a full calendar year, and any changes are generally favorable with regard to the amount of extra help. Table 11–2 summarizes how people qualify for the extra help.

Likewise, people who receive SSI benefits automatically qualify for a full calendar year. They are determined eligible based on data CMS receives from SSA. People who do not

Table 11–2 How People Qualify for Extra Help

Persons with Medicare	How to qualify	Data obtained from what sources?	Can changes occur during the year?
Those with Medicaid benefits • Full Medicaid benefits • Medicare savings program	You are automatically qualified	Your state's files and records	• Qualify for a full calendar year • For the most part only favorable changes will occur
Supplemental security income benefits	You are automatically qualified	Social Security Administration	• Qualify for a full calendar year • For the most part only favorable changes will occur
No Medicaid or supplemental security income benefits	Must apply	Almost all is obtained from the Social Security Administration or your state's files and records	• Some events can impact your status through the year • Extra help can increase, decrease, or be terminated

have Medicaid or receive SSI benefits must apply for the extra help with SSA or their state. Some events, such as marriage, divorce, or separation, can impact the person's extra help status during the year. The amount of extra help can increase, decrease, or terminate.

The coverage gap—"donut hole."   There are things that you can do to reduce your drug costs during the gap and possibly avoid the gap altogether. Under the defined standard benefit in 2006, the coverage gap—for plans that have one—begins after people reach $2,250 in total drug costs. This is called the initial coverage limit, and includes the total cost of the drug, not just what your "true out-of-pocket" (TrOOP) costs are. The TrOOP costs are used to determine the amount of money that you have spent that will determine the additional benefits you are eligible for in the Medicare Part D program. After reaching the initial coverage limit, people pay

100% of their drug costs in the gap until their TrOOP costs total $3,600. Once you spend $3,600 out-of-pocket for covered drug costs during the year, they pay 5% (or a small co-payment of $2 for generic or preferred drugs and $5 for all other drugs) for the rest of the calendar year. This is called catastrophic coverage, and it could start even sooner in some plans. These amounts can change each year. They also vary from plan to plan. During the coverage gap, it is important for you to keep using your prescription drug plan card since:

- The plan has negotiated prices that are generally lower than you can obtain normally from your retail pharmacy, and
- Money spent on covered drugs counts toward TrOOP determination.

Plans track will track your cost spending and will calculate when the coverage gap ends for you.

Best price. If a network pharmacy has better cash price on a covered drug, which is expected to happen rarely, the member may purchase the drug without using his or her Part D card. The cost can count toward total drug spending and TrOOP, but the person must submit documentation to the plan.

If the person finds the drug at a better cash price at a non-network pharmacy, money spent may count toward TrOOP, if the non-network pharmacy usage meets the coverage guidelines when the person:

- Cannot reasonably be expected to obtain such drugs at a network pharmacy; and
- Does not access covered Part D drugs at an out-of-network pharmacy on a routine basis.

Generic drugs. Another option during the gap is switching to generic or less-expensive brand-name drugs, which will reduce co-payments and help maximize savings. Also, switching to generic or less expensive brand-name drugs initially may help a person avoid reaching the gap. In addition, as noted earlier in the book, you can explore other assistance available, including

- The Part D low-income subsidy (extra help)
- State Pharmacy Assistance Programs (SPAPs)
- AIDS Drug Assistance Programs
- Charities in your area
- Patient Assistance Programs (PAPs) from pharmaceutical manufacturers
- Employer/group health plans

State Assistance Plans and Medicare Part D

This past summer, Pennsylvania lawmakers approved a bill that paved the way for the merger of two state prescription drug assistance plans with the Medicare drug benefit. Under the bill, the PACE and PACENET programs — plans that cover low-income Pennsylvanians 65 and older — would pay certain costs for beneficiaries participating in the Medicare drug benefit and provide coverage under the so-called "donut hole" or gap in coverage in the Medicare drug benefit. The legislation strengthened the ability to help PACE and PACENET beneficiaries enroll in the Medicare drug benefit and allow the state to pay monthly premiums for such beneficiaries' enrollment. Some members could qualify for federal subsidies that would cover the cost of joining Part D, slightly lowering their co-pays. Other members, however, could pay more through the Medicare drug benefit.

TrOOP

Not all payments provided by these other sources will count toward a person's TrOOP costs. Payments that will count toward a person's true out-of-pocket (TrOOP) costs include those made by:

- The plan member
- The person's family members or other individuals
- SPAPs—state pharmacy assistance programs
- The extra help (low-income subsidy)
- Charities
  - Unless established, run, or controlled by a current or former employer or union
  - May include Patient Assistance Programs (PAPs), including manufacturer-sponsored PAPs, if established as a charity to help pay cost-sharing

The following payments do not count toward TrOOP:

- Group health plans, including employer or union retiree coverage
- Government-funded programs, including TRICARE or VA
- Other third-party payment arrangements

In case of questions about the coverage gap and what payments will count toward TrOOP:

- Call the plan
- Call your pharmacy
- Visit www.cms.hhs.gov
- Call 1-800-MEDICARE (1-800-633-4227)
- Or call your State Medical Assistance Office

Changes in Formulary Coverage

CMS has instructed Part D plans to not change their therapeutic categories and classes in a formulary other than at the beginning of each plan year, except to account for new therapeutic uses and newly approved Part D drugs. A plan year is a calendar year, January – December. After March 1, 2006, Part D plans could make maintenance changes to their formularies, such as replacing brand-name with new generic drugs or modifying formularies as a result of new information on drug safety or effectiveness. Those changes must be made in accordance with the prescribed approval procedures and following 60 days notice to CMS, SPAPs, prescribing physicians, network pharmacies, pharmacists, and affected members.

Removing drugs from the market.   Part D plans are not required to obtain CMS approval or give 60 days notice when removing formulary drugs that have been withdrawn from the market by either the FDA or a product manufacturer. As noted earlier in the book, beginning on January 1, 2007, Medicare will no longer cover prescription drugs used to treat erectile dysfunction. Medicaid was prohibited from covering erectile dysfunction drugs effective January 1, 2006.

Protection for you.   CMS has issued guidance to Medicare drug plans indicating that no plan members will be subject to a discontinuation or reduction in coverage of the drugs they are currently using. Exceptions can be made in the case of availability of a new generic version of the drug or new FDA or clinical information. CMS expects Part D plans to continue to comply with this policy in 2007 and subsequent plan years, and to include such assurances in their future bids and contracts.

Coverage Determination

A coverage determination is the initial decision made by a plan about the benefits a plan member is entitled to receive or the amount, if any, a member is required to pay for a benefit. An exception request is one type of coverage determination request.

Other examples of a coverage determination include when a plan decides whether or not a person

- Has satisfied a prior authorization requirement—such as having a certain level of functioning or a specific diagnosis for a drug to be covered.

- Has met a step-therapy requirement to have a more expensive drug covered by trying the generic alternative first.
- A person requests more than a 30 day supply of a drug, and the plan initially says no due to quantity limits. You can appeal this decision and seek to obtain 90 days supply—just as you can with a mail order pharmacy participating in the Medicare Part D program.

For example, a person can obtain a drug with a prior authorization (PA) requirement in one of two ways. The person can either (1) satisfy the PA by meeting the requirement set by the plan, or (2) request and be granted an exception to the requirement, based on medical necessity.

If the coverage determination is unfavorable, there may be up to five levels of appeals available. Appeals can be standard or expedited depending on the circumstances, which we'll discuss in a few minutes.

Approvals by you or your authorized representative. The plan member can appeal a Medicare drug plan's unfavorable decision. A representative appointed by the person with Medicare, such as a doctor or family member, may request a coverage determination or an appeal. An appointment of representation form or letter must be filed with the plan sponsor. A person who is an authorized representative (such as a person with power of attorney) may also request a coverage determination or appeal.

In addition to the plan member or appointed representative, your doctor also can request expedited or standard coverage determinations or expedited redeterminations. For other requests, the prescribing physician would need to be an appointed representative. Others can assist people with form completion, gathering evidence, letter writing, etc. A coverage determination can be requested orally or in writing:

- Plans must accept written requests in all cases, but may accept oral requests for standard cases.

- Plans must accept oral requests for expedited coverage determinations and expedited redeterminations.

You or your doctor and the forms required. Two versions of a model coverage determination request form are available, one for use by the plan member, and one for use by the provider. Please see Chapter 7 for copies of both of these forms. Plans may use or modify the model forms and must accept any written request. As we mentioned earlier, an exception request is a type of coverage determination request. There are two types of exceptions including tiering exceptions and formulary exceptions. The criteria for an exception request are established in regulation, and plans may set additional criteria. Exception requests require a supporting statement from the physician, which may be submitted orally or in writing. A supporting statement is not required for other types of coverage determinations. Approved exceptions are valid for refills for the remainder of the plan year, as long as

- You remains enrolled in the plan
- Your physician continues to prescribe the drug
- The drug remains safe for treating the your condition

Yearly Notification

At the end of the plan year the plan will notify members of coverage for the following year. People may need to consider switching to a drug on their plan's formulary, requesting another exception, or changing plans during the Annual Coordinated Election Period. Unlike an approved exception, which is valid for the remainder of the plan year, satisfying a prior authorization requirement may not be valid for the rest of the year. If a person satisfies a plan's prior authorization requirement, it is generally only valid for the number of refills written in the prescription.

Plans must respond promptly. Medicare prescription drug plans have 72 hours to respond to a standard coverage determination request, and 24 hours to respond to an expedited coverage determination request. A request can be considered expedited if applying the standard timeframe will affect your:

- Life or health or
- Ability to regain maximum function

If the doctor indicates or supports medical necessity, the claim must be expedited. If the plan member indicates medical necessity, then the plan will make a decision whether or not to expedite the determination. The clock starts when the plan receives the doctor's supporting statement (exception request) or when the plan receives the request (other coverage determinations). If the plan fails to meet the timeframes, the plan must forward the case to the Part D qualified independent contractor (QIC), which is the independent review entity (IRE), and the request will skip over the first level of appeal (redetermination). The Part D QIC is MAXIMUS; contact information can be found at www.medicarepartdappeals.com on the web.

Level of appeals.   You will receive information about your plan appeal procedures when you enroll in a plan. Appeal requests generally must be made in writing.

- Appeal to the plan (redetermination)—Must be requested within 60 calendar days from the date of receiving the unfavorable decision in writing unless the plan accepts requests by phone. A person can call or write for an expedited request for coverage. The plan has seven days from when it receives a standard request, or 72 hours for an expedited request, to notify the person of its decision.
- Review by an independent review entity—Must be made in writing within 60 days from the date of receiving the plan's unfavorable appeal decision. The IRE has seven days for a standard request, or 72 hours for an ex-

pedited coverage request, to notify the person of its decision.

- Hearing with an administrative law judge (ALJ)—Must be made in writing within 60 days from the date of receiving the unfavorable IRE decision. The projected value of the denied coverage must be $110 or more.
- Review by the Medicare Appeals Council—Must be made in writing within 60 days from the date of receiving the unfavorable ALJ decision.
- Review by a Federal court—If the MAC agrees with the plan's decision, the person can file a written request for review by a Federal court. To receive a review by a Federal court, the amount must be $1,090 or greater.

The minimum amounts for ALJ hearings and federal court review are determined annually, and appeals may be placed together to meet their needs.

Your Personal Health Information and Privacy

There are circumstances under which a health plan, such as a Medicare drug plan, may disclose relevant protected health information (PHI) to someone who is assisting the plan member, specifically regarding the drug benefit. It is important to note that these health plans are permitted, but not required, to make these disclosures under the following conditions:

1. Plans may disclose relevant PHI to those identified by the plan member as being involved in his or her care or payment, such as helping to resolve a Part D enrollment issue:
   - Family member or other relative
   - Close personal friend
   - CMS staff, Congressional staff, or other person providing assistance

2. Plans may disclose relevant PHI when:
- The member is present and agrees/does not object or the plan reasonably infers from the circumstances that he or she does not object.
- The member is not present or is incapacitated; the plan may exercise its professional judgment to determine whether disclosure is in the member's best interests.

Please see Appendix F for a brochure from the United States Department of Health and Human Services that describes what your rights are related to your personal health information.

Initial Enrollment Periods

On May 15, 2006, the first Initial Enrollment Period ended for people entitled to Medicare in January 2006 or earlier. All people who become entitled to Medicare after January 2006 have a seven-month Initial Enrollment Period (IEP) for Part D:

- You can apply three months before your month of Medicare eligibility. Coverage will begin on the date you become eligible.
- You apply in your month of eligibility, in which case their Part D coverage will begin on the first of the following month.
- Or you can also apply during the three months after your month of eligibility, with coverage beginning the first of the month after the month they apply.

Some groups of people who become entitled to Medicare will be enrolled in a Part D plan by CMS unless they join a plan on their own.

Where Else Might You Obtain Help in Enrolling?

Your United States congressman or United States Senators have local field offices in the state where you live. There are people in these offices that can help you with enrollment questions, or to help you if you have problems with a particular plan or what you are being told by the plan. These offices are set up to serve you, I would encourage you to seek help from them should you need assistance.

Enrollment materials.   People who are new to Medicare and enroll in a plan, or who are enrolled in a plan by CMS, can expect to receive an enrollment letter and membership materials from the plan. The materials will contain an identification card and customer service information including a toll-free phone number and website. People who are taking a drug that is not on their new plan formulary can generally get a 30-day transition supply. This gives them time to work with their prescribing physician to find a different drug that is on the plan's formulary. If an acceptable alternative drug is not available, they or their physician can request an exception from the plan, and denied requests can be appealed. This is also what people can expect when they join a new Part D plan during the Annual Coordinated Election Period or a Special Enrollment Period.

Annual Coordinated Election Period (AEP).   In most cases, once people have enrolled in a Medicare drug plan, they will remain in that plan until the end of the plan year. They will be able to switch plans or disenroll during the Annual Coordinated Election Period (AEP), November 15 to December 31 each year.

Like dual eligibles, people in a Medicare Savings Program and people who live in a long-term care facility have a continuous Special Enrollment Period. They can change plans at any time and will have the new drug coverage effective the first of the following month.

Others facilitated into a plan by CMS if they did not choose one on their own (people who applied and qualified for the extra help and people with Medicare and SSI-only) can switch plans or disenroll once before the end of the plan year.

Extra help. When people with Medicare who are already enrolled in a Medicare drug plan are found eligible for the extra help, the plan is notified. The plan will refund the premiums and cost-sharing assistance the members would have received, back to the month they were found to be eligible. Plans are randomly chosen from those with premiums at or below the regional benchmark. CMS chooses plans with premiums at or below the regional benchmark so that people who are entitled to the full extra help subsidy pay no premium. Those entitled to a partial subsidy will pay a reduced or no premium. People who are already in a Medicare Advantage Plan will be enrolled in the same plan with prescription drug coverage (MA-PD), if offered by the MA organization.

Automatic enrolling. CMS will notify people who will be enrolled in a Medicare Prescription Drug Plan. People who are being auto-enrolled receive a letter on yellow paper.

Those being facilitated receive a letter on green paper, in one of two versions—full subsidy or partial subsidy, depending on the subsidy level of the extra help. The facilitated enrollment letter includes a list of the plans in that region that are at or below the regional benchmark premium, so people can look for other plans that meets their needs. Medicare Advantage Plans send the notice when they will be enrolling one of their members in an MA-PD. In Spring 2005, CMS began determining individuals eligible for extra help for all of 2006. Starting in August, 2006, CMS will redetermine individuals for calendar year 2007 on the basis of their continued eligibility as a full or partial dual eligible or SSI recipient. These changes will be effective January 1, 2007.

People who are currently automatically eligible for 2006 will continue to qualify for the extra help through December 2006. If they are no longer eligible, their automatic status will end on December 31, 2006.

Notification. After CMS completes the redetermination process for people who automatically qualified for the extra help in 2006, notices will be mailed. People who will no longer automatically qualify for extra help in 2007 will receive a letter from CMS with an extra help application from SSA. People who will have a change in their co-payment level between 2006 and 2007 (e.g. from $1/$3 to $0 or from $0 to $2.15/$5.35) will receive a letter from CMS. These letters will be mailed in September 2006. People who will continue to automatically qualify for extra help at the same cost-sharing level will not receive a letter from CMS or an application from SSA. (If people who lose their automatic eligibility later become re-entitled to Medicaid benefits or SSI, CMS will mail them a new letter informing them that they now automatically qualify for extra help.)

People who apply and qualify for the extra help are required to reestablish their eligibility each year with the agency that made the initial determination, either SSA or the state Medicaid program office. For people who applied and qualified for the extra help in 2005, the initial determination will be in effect for all of 2006. (However, people who applied and were denied can apply again if their circumstances change.) For people who apply for the first time in 2006, the initial determination stays in effect for up to a year. After the initial determination, SSA and the states set their respective redetermination timeframes, with states basing the timeframes on their Medicaid rules. However, SSA and states use the same set of national standards to determine eligibility. All decisions may be appealed, including denials, effective dates, and partial subsidies, with the agency that was responsible for the decision. SSA is required to make a redetermination for each individual who qualifies for extra help within 12 months of their initial eligibility.

SSA is sent a letter in late August 2006 to all people who applied and qualified for extra help by the end of April 2006 and who have not become automatically eligible. (Note: anyone approved for the extra help by SSA after April 30 will not have subsidy eligibility redetermined until 2007.) The letter will ask the individual if his/her income and resources are still below or within certain limits and instruct him or her to reply

Summary and Next Steps

if there is a change. Individuals who return the initial letter saying there has been a change will receive a redetermination form, which they must complete and return to SSA within 30 days. Any change will be effective January 1, 2007. SSA will also redetermine eligibility on a random sample of cases for quality assurance purposes. For each set of sample cases, all factors affecting eligibility and/or whether a person should receive a full or partial subsidy may be verified by contacting the enrollee and also using other information sources, for example, employers to verify wage information.

Changes affecting your extra help situation. Eligibility for the extra help can also change throughout the year if SSA receives a report from a person with Medicare or from another source (e.g. data exchange of reports of death) of a change in eligibility based on

- Marriage
- Married couple resumes living together after having been separated
- Death of spouse, who lived in same home
- Divorce
- Separation (i.e., person or spouse moves out of the household and the couple is no longer living together, this is unless the separation is a temporary absence).
- An annulment of a marriage.

Upon receipt of such a report, SSA will send a redetermination form. The person must return the completed form to SSA within 90 days of the date of the form. If the person does not return the redetermination form, the subsidy will be terminated. Any change in the person's subsidy will be effective the month following the month of your report.

Special enrollment periods (SEPs). There are a number of situations when people have a Special Enrollment Period and can add, change, or drop Medicare drug coverage.

- People who involuntarily lose their creditable prescription drug coverage have 60 days from the date of termination or notice of termination, whichever is later, to enroll in a Medicare drug plan. Creditable drug coverage is coverage that is as good as Medicare prescription drug coverage.
- People who get Medicare and Medicaid benefits (i.e., dual eligibles) or help from their state paying for their Medicare premiums (Medicare Savings Programs) may enroll in a Part D plan or switch plans at any time, with the new plan effective the first day of the following month.
- People who lose dual eligibility status have three months to change their Part D plan.
- People who permanently move out of their plan's service area have up to two months after moving to enroll in a new Part D plan.
- People who move into a long-term care facility, like a nursing home, can enroll in or change plans at any time, with the new plan effective the first day of the following month. They also have two months after moving out to enroll in or change plans.
- People who are eligible for the extra help and were facilitated into a Part D plan have at least one opportunity to switch out of that plan during the plan year.
- People found eligible for the extra help after May 15, 2006, may enroll in a plan through December 31, 2006, using a Special Enrollment Period.

Losing Coverage Through No Fault of Your Own

Here is an example of the Special Enrollment Period for people with Medicare who lose creditable drug coverage through no fault of their own. In this example (Figure 11–1), the person receives notice on July 15 that his/her creditable drug coverage will end on August 31. The SEP for loss of creditable coverage is 60 days from either the loss of coverage

Example of Creditable Coverage SEP

SEP = 60 days from <u>either</u> loss of coverage OR date notice received, whichever is later.

Begins when individual advised of loss = e.g., July 15

Example: SEP ends October 30 = 60 days from coverage ending is October 30 > date of July 15 notice

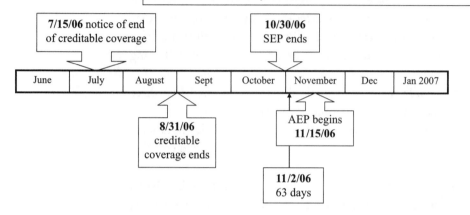

Figure 11–1   Example of Creditable Coverage SEP

or the date the notice is received, whichever is later. In this case, August 31, the date of the loss of coverage, is later, so the person has 60 days—September 1 through October 30—to sign up for a prescription drug plan using the SEP. If people enroll in a Part D plan with no gap in creditable coverage of 63 days or more, they will not incur a penalty for the period without coverage.

Special Enrollment Periods

CMS has added two new SEPs for people with Medicare including those who lived in an area affected by Hurricane Katrina, and those who are found eligible for the extra help after May 15, 2006. CMS will grant all Hurricane Katrina evacuees a Special Enrollment Period (SEP) to give them more time to change Medicare prescription drug plans in 2006. Individuals will be considered "evacuees" and eligible for this SEP if they lived in certain ZIP codes, as identified by the Federal Emergency Management Agency, at the time of the hurricane (August 2005). The special enrollment period means that Katrina evacuees will be able to switch plans, including Medicare prescription drug plans, at any time through December 31, 2006. To determine if an individual is eligible for this SEP, Medicare plans must first attempt to obtain proof that the individual resided in an affected ZIP code (e.g., driver's license, utility bills, etc.). If the individual is unable to provide such proof, the plan must accept the person's attestation that he or she resided in an affected ZIP code. Persons with Medicare who are found eligible for the extra help between May 15, 2006 and December 31, 2006, receive a SEP to enroll in a Medicare drug plan if they are not already in one. The SEP lasts from the time they are found eligible until December 31, 2006. In both of these situations, eligible individuals will not incur a penalty if they enroll in a Medicare drug plan by December 31, 2006. All people with Medicare can join, switch, or drop Medicare drug plans during the Annual Coordinated Election Period (AEP). The next AEP will be November 15 through December 31, 2006. Changes will be effective January 1, 2007. There will be an AEP from November 15 through December 31 every year, with changes effective the following January 1.

Notice of Plan Change Requirements

Each year, both stand-alone prescription drug plans (PDPs) and Medicare Advantage plans with prescription drug coverage (MA-PDs) are required to send an annual notice of change to all plan members. In 2006, the letter must be sent, along with a Summary of Benefits and a copy of the formulary for the upcoming year, in time to arrive no later than October 31, 2006. The letter will explain any changes to their current plan, including changes to the monthly premium and cost-sharing information such as co-payments or coinsurance. In addition to the Initial Enrollment Period for Part D, and the Annual Coordinated Election Period each year, people with Medicare can join a Medicare Advantage Plan during an Open Enrollment Period each year. People can join a new plan or switch plans. (Note that Other Medicare Plans follow different rules.)

- In 2006, the Open Enrollment Period was January 1 through June 30.
- In 2007 and every year after, the Open Enrollment Period will be January 1 through March 31.
- Changes will be effective the first of the month after the person joined or switched plans.

The MA Open Enrollment Period can be used to switch to a different type of plan, but it cannot be used to change whether or not the person is enrolled in Medicare prescription drug coverage.

Options During Enrollment Periods

An enrollment period gives people one opportunity to join, switch, or drop plans. This applies to the Initial Enrollment Period, Special Enrollment Periods, the Annual Coordinated Election Period, and the Medicare Advantage Open Enrollment Period. Once the change has taken effect, that enrollment period is over for that person. If someone disenrolls from a plan, that uses the person's one opportunity for that enrollment period. It is important to remember that enrolling in a new drug plan will automatically disenroll people from their current Medicare plan. This includes individuals who are enrolled in most Medicare Advantage Plans. People do not need to request disenrollment from the current plan unless they want to drop Medicare drug coverage completely. In that case, the individual must request disenrollment by contacting the current plan or 1-800-MEDICARE (1-800-633-4227). TTY users should call 1-877-486-2048.

Special Circumstances

If someone disenrolls from a plan and the change becomes effective, that uses the person's one opportunity to join, switch, or drop plans. However, if the person enrolls in a new plan with the same effective date, the new enrollment will be processed. But people who wait and do not apply to join a new plan until the following month will not be able to enroll until their next enrollment period. If a person does not have creditable coverage, this means that he or she also may be subject to a late enrollment penalty.

Penalty or Not

You already know that people who do not enroll in Part D at their first opportunity may have to pay a penalty to enroll later. Most people who do not join a Medicare drug plan during their Initial Enrollment Period will have to pay an additional premium amount for every month they wait to enroll, unless they have other coverage that is at least as good as standard Medicare prescription drug coverage. This is called "creditable" coverage. To avoid a penalty, people must not have any gaps in creditable coverage of 63 or more consecutive days.

People with this penalty will have to pay it as long as they have Medicare prescription drug coverage. To encourage people with limited income and resources to get drug coverage, CMS will not require plans to collect a late enrollment penalty for the rest of 2006 for all people receiving the extra help—either full or partial subsidy—or who lived in areas affected by Hurricane Katrina. This is in addition to granting the ongoing Special Enrollment Period for 2006 for these people, which we discussed earlier, that allows them to enroll in a Part D plan for 2006 at any time before the end of the year. If these individuals enroll in 2006 and stay continuously enrolled in a Part D plan, they will never have to pay a penalty. Those who drop drug coverage after 2006 may be subject to a penalty if they reenroll at a later date. If these individuals wait until after 2006 to enroll, they will be subject to the late enrollment penalty if they have any gap of 63 continuous days or longer in their creditable prescription drug coverage. The penalty will include months in 2006 if they were eligible for Part D and did not have creditable coverage.

Changes in the Prescription Plan Finder for 2007

The Medicare Prescription Drug Plan Finder is being updated to have a "cleaner" look and feel and will require less scrolling by users. (The same data will be available.) Beginning October 12, 2006, information on the 2007 drug plans will be available. From October 12 through December 31, 2006, people will have access to both 2006 and 2007 plan year data. Beginning November 15, performance metrics for plans that existed in 2006 will be available within the tool. The Medicare Personal Plan Finder is undergoing a major redesign, including being renamed, and will be more integrated with the drug plan finder. An authenticated search option is being added to Personal Plan Finder (just like the drug plan finder), which allows the system to query the Medicare Beneficiary Database and display the current plan enrollment information.

Summary of Considerations and Next Steps

There has been a lot presented in this chapter. There are some basic things that you need to decide upon:

Cost

This includes the premium amount, the deductible, and the co-payments required before higher levels of support kick in for you. Co-payments may be different for generic drugs, brand name drugs, and other brand name preferred drugs. There is a need for you to consider many factors presented here in the book.

Formulary Coverage

This coverage will vary from plan to plan. Your drugs may not be covered in each of the plans. The formulary finder will allow you to see what is available in your state, and how many of your drugs are covered. The nice thing about this formulary finder that CMS provides allows you to see if a generic is available for drugs that you are required to take.

Coverage Gap.   There is a coverage gap that some of you will need to consider. Some of the plans provide some coverage for the drugs that you take in this gap ("donut hole"). Here your true out of pocket (TrOOP) costs come into play.

Convenience

Can you obtain your medicines at your regular pharmacy? This is an important issue for many people. Check to see if your pharmacy participates in one or more of the plans that you are considering

Peace of Mind

It may be to your benefit to sign up for a plan. One never knows how many drugs that you might take in the future.

Creditable Coverage

See if the coverage that you have now is better than what you might have with the Medicare Part D Plan. Remember, if you lose your creditable coverage for a reason out of your control, you will qualify for signing up for Medicare Part D. If you have Medigap prescription coverage from a company, generally this will not be as good as what you can obtain through the Medicare Part D program.

What Happens If You Move During the Year to Another State?

The following also applies if you move within a state with differing coverage in different parts of the state. If you move, you will have up to four months to select a new plan. You must however, notify the plan that you currently have and let them know that you are moving to a different permanent address.

Summary and Next Steps

What If I Am Not Happy with My Plan?

If you are not satisfied with your current Medicare Part D prescription drug plan, please know that you can change plans during the next enrollment period. Outside of this enrollment period, it will be difficult for you to change plans. If you qualify for extra help, you will be able to switch plans. Do not feel that you are "stuck" with a plan, if it does not work for you, switch to one that does. You owe this to yourself.

State Resources That Can Help You

State health insurance assistance programs (SHIPS) are state helping agencies that have provided help with Medicare Part D questions, dilemmas, and problems for thousands of Medicare recipients. Personnel with SHIPs in numerous states are concerned about the enrollment periods for Medicare Part D. These periods are at the end of the year during holiday seasons. I would encourage you to seek help months in advance to start obtaining the help that you need and deserve. One problem that has come to light with beneficiaries already with Medicare Part D coverage is overcharging for their drugs at pharmacies. This has especially occurred with individuals in the LIS category who are dual eligible and have been charged too much.

Types of Problems That Have Occurred

With any new governmental program, problems can occur. If you experience any of the following, contact Medicare, your state SHIP agency, or your Congressmen or Senator for assistance:

Incorrect premium deduction. This has happened and in some cases due to delays, several premiums will be deducted at the same time. This may place a burden on your finances.

Overcharging at the pharmacy. The computer systems involved with the program do not always provide timely information to pharmacists. Please double check the amounts that you have been charged for your drugs. If are eligible for extra assistance because of your income, dual eligibility for both Medicare and Medicaid, or have LIS assistance you should be charged minimally for your drugs or nothing in most cases.

Prior authorization hassles.   Some clients have indicated that they have to go through the process of prior authorization for their drugs monthly. If you have received approval for your drugs, you should have this approval for the balance of the year. You do not have to go through this process each month. You will have to go through this at the start of the next year, but the approval is good for the balance of the year in which it has been granted to you.

Doctors not being willing to fill out the prior authorization paperwork.   This is regrettable, your doctor should do this for you—it is for your benefit! Be insistent, unless there is a good reason for you not receiving the drug. There may be instances where your drug has been taken off the market and is just not available any longer. Some drugs to treat erectile dysfunction will not be covered beginning January 2007. Also some drugs are not covered under Medicare Part D at all (e.g., Valium®).

Medicare Advantage plans.   Individuals have expressed frustration with Medicare Advantage plans and not understanding what the plan covers and what services they provide. This has been mentioned previously in this book

Deceitful marketing practices.   Some plans have marketed life insurance or long-term care insurance plans alongside Medicare Part D Plans. People affected assume that these other programs are government sponsored parts of Medicare —they are not!

Spouses of individuals in nursing homes.   People with coverage under employer plans for husband and wife who are admitted to nursing homes and automatically are enrolled in Medicare Part D. The spouse still living at home loses employer coverage, and is not eligible for other coverage as well without paying a penalty.

Nursing home residents. People helping within SHIPs do not counsel nursing home residents. If you are in a nursing home, and need some help the nursing home should be providing information to the client on where to turn for help if there are problems.

Consider all of the above, think about what is best for you, and please make the most informed decision that you can. You owe it to yourself to get the most from all the Medicare programs you participate in, including this new Medicare Part D Plan.

References

1. CMS press release, *"More than 100,000 now in Pilot Medicare Health Support Programs: Programs Help Beneficiaries with Chronic Conditions,"* February 3, 2006
2. Part of Medicare Prescription Drug, Improvement, and Modernization Act of 2003, Section 721.
3. www.cms.hhs.gov/center/ombudsman.asp
   How Medicare's Beneficiary Ombudsman is Working For You, CMS Pub.11173, November 2005

Other Sources Used

Medicare Prescription Drug, Improvement, and Modernization Act of 2003, Section 923

Model forms for use in requesting formulary exceptions or appeals and coverage determination requests: www.cms.hhs.gov/Prescription-DrugCovContra/06_RxContracting_EnrollmentAppeals.asp

General Summary of the Issues Related to Medicare Part D Medicare Prescription Drug Benefit Information

People with Medicare Must Make an Important Decision This Year

Medicare added a new prescription drug benefit in 2006. Everyone with Medicare must decide if they want to enroll. Choosing to delay enrolling until a later time will result in higher premiums.

How Will the Medicare Prescription Benefit Be Offered?

Medicare will contract with private companies to offer prescription drug plans. To receive prescription benefits you will select one of these plans. There are two types of plans:

1. You can choose to receive your medical benefits from the traditional Medicare program and receive prescription drug coverage through a Prescription Drug Plan (PDP).

OR

2. You can join a Medicare Advantage plan. Medicare Advantage plans provide another way to receive your Medicare benefits, including the new drug benefit. Medicare Advantage plans can be a Health Maintenance Organization (HMO), Preferred Provider Organization (PPO) or a Private-Fee-For-Service plan (PFFS).

The plans will start January 1, 2006. There will be several to choose from in each state. If you join a plan, you will pay a monthly premium (around $32 in 2006) and pay some of the cost of your prescriptions. How much you pay, what drugs are covered, and which pharmacy you use will vary depending on the plan you choose.

Who Is Eligible?

You are eligible for the Medicare prescription drug benefit if you are enrolled in Medicare Part A and/or Part B.

When Can I Enroll?

You can enroll anytime between November 15, 2005 and May 15, 2006. Join by December 31, 2005, and your Medicare prescription drug coverage will begin on January 1, 2006. If you join after that, your coverage will begin the first day of the month after you enroll. New Medicare enrollees will be able to enroll in a prescription drug plan when they enroll in Medicare.

Delaying Enrollment

If you are eligible to join a plan and you do not join a plan by May 15, 2006, and you do not have an existing drug plan that is at least as good as the Medicare prescription drug coverage, then you will pay a higher premium when you do enroll.

How Does the Medicare Prescription Drug Coverage Work?

This is how a basic prescription drug plan will work in 2006:

- You will pay a monthly premium of about $32.20. Some plans will charge more, other less.
- You will pay the first $250 of your drug costs each year. This is called a deductible.
- After you pay the deductible, Medicare will pay 75% of the next $2,000 of your drug costs. You pay 25% of these costs or $500.
- After total drug costs reach $2,250, you will pay 100% of drug costs on the next $2,850. Once your out-of-pocket drug costs, not including premiums, reach $3,600 ($250 deductible + $500 coinsurance + $2,850 coverage gap), Medicare will start paying 95% of your drug costs. (Please see chart below)
- Some plans may offer additional benefits that would increase premium costs

Basic Prescription Benefit			
Your Drug Costs	You Pay	Medicare Pays	Your Total Out-of-Pocket Costs Per Year*
$0–$265	100% ($265)	$0	$265
$265–$2,400	25% ($600)	75% ($1,800)	$865
$2,400–$5,451.25	100% ($3,051.25)	$0	$3,916.25
Over $5,451.25	5%	95%	$3,916.25 + 5% of costs above $5,451.25

*Does not include premium costs

How Do I Enroll?

Beginning in October 2005, you can compare plans with an on-line tool at www.medicare.gov—*Finding* a *Medicare Prescription Drug Plan.* After choosing a plan you will enroll with that private company. If you have trouble making a decision,

Appendix A

your state agency on aging can help you compare your choices and enroll in a plan that meets your needs.

If you have a Medicare supplement plan with drug coverage you will get a notice before November 15, 2005 from your insurance company. It will explain how your plan will work with Medicare prescription drug coverage and your options.

What If I Have a Medicare Supplement with Drug Coverage?

If you have a Medicare supplement policy H, I or J with drug coverage you must decide if you want to keep it or choose a different policy.

- If you keep the original H, I or J plan with drug coverage and do not enroll in a prescription drug plan, you will pay a higher premium if you decide to enroll at a later date.
- If you decide to enroll in a prescription drug plan during the initial enrollment period, you can keep plan H, I or J with the prescription drug coverage removed or choose a different Medicare supplement plan. Your choices will be plans A, B, C, F, K or L (K and L are new plans that will be offered beginning in 2006).

What If I Have an Employer/Union Plan with Drug Coverage?

Your employer/union will notify you before November 15, 2005 if your plan's prescription benefit is at *least* as *good* as a Medicare prescription drug plan.

- If your employer drug plan is as good as or has better coverage than Part D, you can stay with that plan and join a Medicare prescription drug plan later with no extra cost.
- If your current prescription drug plan offers less coverage than Part D, you can keep your plan and add a

Medicare drug plan to give you more complete coverage.

OR

- If you stay on your current drug plan with less coverage than Part D and decide to join a Medicare prescription drug plan later (after May 15, 2005), you will pay at least 1 % more for every month you waited to get a Medicare prescription drug plan.

What If I Am Enrolled in Medicare and My Supplemental Insurance Does Not Have Prescription Drug Coverage?

- If you are enrolled in a Medicare supplement that does not have prescription drug coverage, you need to carefully consider your Medicare prescription drug plan options.
- You can keep your supplement and enroll in a Medicare prescription drug plan.
- You can keep your current coverage and not enroll in a Medicare prescription drug plan, but you will have to pay at least 1 % more for every month you waited to get a Medicare prescription drug plan if you choose to enroll at a later time.
- You can choose to receive your Medicare benefits, including prescription drugs, through a Medicare Advantage Plan (HMO, PPO, PFFS) instead of through traditional Medicare and a supplement.

What If I Am Enrolled in a Medicare Advantage Plan?

If your Medicare Advantage plan provides drug coverage at least as good as the Medicare prescription drug benefit you are not eligible to enroll in a prescription drug plan. Your Medicare Advantage plan will notify you before November 15, 2006 if your coverage is "as good as" the Medicare prescription drug benefit and what your options are for enrolling in a prescription drug plan.

What If I Have Military Service or Veterans Prescription Drug Benefits?

These programs will notify you if they are at least as good as the Medicare prescription drug benefit and what your options are for enrolling in the Medicare prescription drug benefit.

What If I Cannot Afford a Prescription Drug Plan?

People with limited income and resources will qualify for extra help paying their premium and for some of the cost of their prescriptions.

Does Medicaid Pay for Your Prescription Drugs?

If you are on Medicare and receiving full Medicaid benefits (including prescription drug coverage) you will automatically get extra help and be enrolled in a prescription drug plan. This replaces your Medicaid drug coverage beginning January 1, 2006. The following table explains what you will pay with the basic Medicare prescription drug plan.

Individuals on Medicare with Medicaid Prescription Benefits		
	Living In a Nursing Hom or Medical Institution	Income Below $9,570 for an Individual; $12,830 for a Couple
Premium	$0	$0
Deductible	$0	$0
Co-payment	$0	$1 for generic prescription, $3 for brand name prescription
Catastrophic Coverage	$0	You pay nothing after your total drug expenses reach $5,100

Do You Have a Limited Income But *Do Not* Qualify for Medicaid Coverage for Your Prescription Drugs?

You may still qualify for extra help with your prescriptions if your income is below $14,355 if you are single and $19,245 if you are married and your assets are below $11,500 for singles and $23,000 for married. The chart below explains the benefits and how you qualify.

People with Medicare and Medicaid without Drug Coverage		
Income	Income Below† $12,920/individual* $17,321/couple*	Income Below $$14,355/individual* $19,245/couple*
Assets	Below $6,000/individual $9,000/couple	Below $11,500/individual 23,000/couple
Premium	$0	premium based upon income
Deductible	$0	$50
Co-payment	$2 for generic prescription, $5 for brand name prescription	15% coinsurance
	You pay nothing after your total drug expenses reach $5,000	$2 for generic prescription; $5 for brand name prescription after drug expenses reach $5,100

*2005 Income Requirement; †Includes individuals enrolled in SSI and Medicare Savings Programs (QMB, SLMB, QI-1)

If you think you qualify for extra help with drug plan costs, you must follow a two-step process:

1. First, you must *apply for the extra help* paying prescription plan costs; contact your local Social Security office after July 1, 2005. Enrollment can be done by mail, telephone or online.
2. Then, you must *enroll in* a *Medicare prescription drug plan* that meets your needs. Enrollment in the plans began November 15, 2005.

When Will I *Get* More Information About the Prescription Drug Plans?

In October, you will be able to compare the benefits of each of the plans at www.medicare.gov - *Finding* a *Medicare Prescription Drug Plan,* 1-800-MEDICARE (1-800-633-4227). TTY users, call 1-877-486-2048.

How Do I Choose a Medicare Prescription Drug Plan?

You should compare the costs of your prescriptions with the benefits provided by each of the plans to make sure you choose a plan that meets your needs. Your state agency on aging can provide personalized help when plan information becomes available in October, 2005.

REMEMBER...

- If you meet the income and asset limits, you may qualify for extra help.
- If you get a letter from your insurance company saying that you do not have to sign up for Part D, KEEP it as proof of coverage.

Source: Jack E. Fincham, Ph.D.
A.W. Jowdy Professor of Pharmacy Care
The University of Georgia
College of Pharmacy
Athens, GA 30602
706-542-5311
jfincham@uga.edu
©All Rights Reserved, November, 2006

The information in this document is current as of November, 2006. Please understand that the information will change in subsequent years. Deductibles will no doubt increase, and expected amounts to be paid before coverage will increase as well.

Websites for Senior Citizen Information

> Specific websites with information of use to seniors, families, and caregivers about Medicare Part D.

Centers for Medicare and Medicaid Services

Information about prescription drug plans and coverage issues:

http://www.cms.hhs.gov/PrescriptionDrugCovGenIn/03_
Resources.asp#TopOfPage

General information about prescription drug coverage:

http://www.cms.hhs.gov/PrescriptionDrugCovGenIn/

Comparing various plans, examining your current plan:

http://www.medicare.gov/MPDPF

Medicare Education

www.medicareeducation.org

Social Security Administration Website

www.ssa.gov

The National Council on Aging

NCOA is a national voice and powerful advocate for public policies that promote vital aging.

http://www.ncoa.org

Access to Benefits Coalition™

Rx access for those who need them most. There are currently more than 70 national non-profit members of the Access to Benefits Coalition™, who share the interest of helping low-income Medicare beneficiaries find the public and private prescription savings programs they need to maintain their health and improve the quality of their lives.

http://www.accesstobenefits.org

Various helpful resources on programs saving money for seniors and their drug use.

www.crbestbuydrugs.org/: contains important information from Consumer Reports about saving money on prescription drugs.

www.ashp.org/pap/: Created by the American Society of Health-System Pharmacists with support from the Health Resources and Services Administration. Provides information on patient assistance programs.

www.eldercare.gov: Run by the U.S. Administration on Aging. Shows drug assistance programs by state. (800) 677-1116.

www.gskforyou.com/index.htm. GlaxoSmithKline Pharmaceutical Company patient assistance website.

www.needymeds.com: Lists information about state programs, discount drug cards, federal poverty guidelines, and patient assistance programs and includes copies of the forms.

www.rxassist.com: Run by Volunteers in Health Care. Allows searches by medicine and manufacturer, and helps find assistance programs nationwide.

www.helpingpatients.org: A resource for patient assistance programs. Run by the Pharmaceutical Research and Manufacturers of America.

www.merckhelps.com. A resource for patient assistance programs. Provided by Merck and Company.

General Health Information Sources

WebMD Health

http://my.webmd.com/medical_information/condition_centers/default.htm

http://my.webmd.com/medical_information/medicare_rx_benefits/default.htm

The Mayo Clinic

http://www.mayoclinic.com/index.cfm

United States government healthfinder affiliated organizations and websites:

http://www.healthfinder.gov/organizations/

Several disease based national organization websites

American Heart Association

http://www.americanheart.org

American Diabetes Association

http://www.diabetes.org

American Cancer Society

http://www.cancer.org

American Lung Association

http://www.lungusa.org

Several websites especially designed for women:

http://www.womens-health.org/consumers.htm

http://www.4woman.gov/

Individual States with Medication Assistance Programs for Seniors with Certain Income Restrictions

Alaska
California
Connecticut
Delaware
Florida
Hawaii
Illinois
Indiana
Kentucky
Maine
Maryland
Massachusetts
Missouri
Montana
Nevada

New Hampshire
New Jersey
New York
North Carolina
Pennsylvania
Rhode Island
South Carolina
Texas
Vermont
Washington
Wisconsin
Wyoming
U.S. Virgin Islands

Adapted from http://www.aarp.org/bulletin/prescription/statebystate .html, accessed August 9, 2006 & Kaiser Family Foundation. Accessed at: http://www.statehealthfacts.org

Petition Process for Formulary Addition and Notification of Noncoverage

Medicare Part D Appeals Process

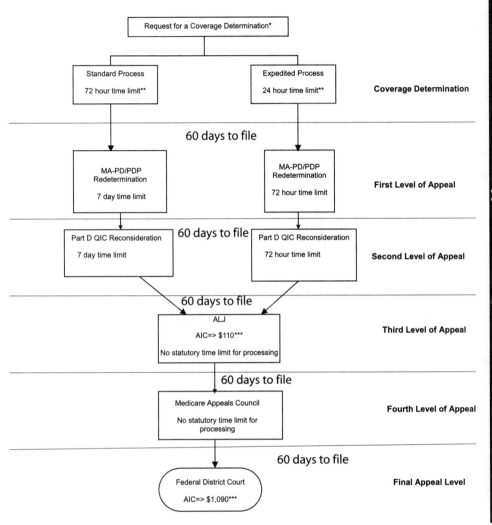

AIC = Amount in controversy
ALJ = Administrative Law Judge
IRE = Independent Review Entity
MA-PD = Medicare Advantage plan that offers Part D benefits
PDP = Prescription Drug Plan

*A request for a coverage determination includes a request for a tiering exception or a formulary exception. A request for a coverage determination may be filed by the enrollee, the enrollee's appointed representative, or the enrollee's physician.

**The adjudication timeframes generally begin when the request is received by the plan sponsor. However, if the request involves an exception request, the adjudication timeframe begins when the plan sponsor receives the physician's supporting statement.

***Starting in 2005, the AIC requirement for an ALJ hearing and Federal District Court will be adjusted in accordance with the medical care component of the consumer price index.

Source: CMS Pub. No. 11195

Websites for More Information About Drugs

Before I list the specific websites I would like to provide here, I want to say a little about websites and information that appears on the internet. Not everything that is on the website provides accurate information. Some of what appears is not worth reading, and certainly is suspect in the accuracy of the materials presented. There is foundation called Health on the Net (HON) that will help guide you to accurate information. The mission of HON is as listed on their website:

> is to guide the growing community of healthcare consumers and providers on the World Wide Web to sound, reliable medical information and expertise. In this way, HON seeks to contribute to better, more accessible and cost-effective health care.

If the website that you are examining has the seal of approval from HON it lets you know that the site has been evaluated for accuracy. HON provides a code of conduct for web information. It can be found at:

http://www.hon.ch/HONcode/Conduct.html

I will recommend only those sites that provide unbiased drug information for consumers. Many websites provide drug information, but also do it for the purposes of encouraging the consumer to purchase medications on-line.

National Library of Medicine and National Institutes of Health

http://www.nlm.nih.gov/medlineplus/druginformation.html

http://medlineplus.gov/esp/

(Both Español and English versions)

The Mayo Clinic

http://www.mayoclinic.com/index.cfm

The Herbal Research Foundation supports a website with comprehensive information about herbs and herbal supplements

http://www.herbs.org/

The United States Food and Drug Administration Websites for Consumer Education and Information

"Consumer Education: What You Should Know About Buying and Using Drug Products"

FDA is committed to providing consumers with information on prescription, generic, and over-the-counter drug products. The Center for Drug Evaluation and Research has developed numerous public service campaigns and announcements to help you make informed decisions about using medicines.

http://www.fda.gov/cder/consumerinfo/DPAdefault.htm

United States FDA website on the dangers of mixing drugs and alcohol

http://www.asyouage.samhsa.gov/Default.aspx

United States FDA website on several drugs which should not be purchased from non-United States sources

http://www.fda.gov/cder/consumerinfo/dontBuyonNet.htm

Consumer Information from Other Government Agencies

Agency for Healthcare Research and Quality

Five Steps to Safer Health Care

http://www.healthfinder.gov/

United States Food and Drug Administration website for information on nutritional supplements.

http://vm.cfsan.fda.gov/~dms/supplmnt.html

www.fda.gov/buyonline: An FDA resource for buying drugs online.

www.fda.gov/cder/consumerinfo/DPAdefault.htm: An FDA resource on medication safety.

Privacy and Health Information Pamphlet Provided by the U.S. Department of Health and Human Services Office of Civil Rights

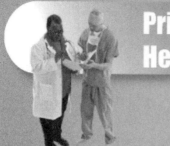

Privacy and Your Health Information

Your Privacy Is Important to All of Us

Most of us feel that our health and medical information is private and should be protected, and we want to know who has this information. Now, Federal law

► Gives you rights over your health information

► Sets rules and limits on who can look at and receive your health information

Your Health Information Is Protected By Federal Law

Who must follow this law?

► Most doctors, nurses, pharmacies, hospitals, clinics, nursing homes, and many other health care providers

► Health insurance companies, HMOs, most employer group health plans

► Certain government programs that pay for health care, such as Medicare and Medicaid

What information is protected?

► Information your doctors, nurses, and other health care providers put in your medical record

► Conversations your doctor has about your care or treatment with nurses and others

► Information about you in your health insurer's computer system

► Billing information about you at your clinic

► Most other health information about you held by those who must follow this law

The Law Gives You Rights Over Your Health Information

Providers and health insurers who are required to follow this law must comply with your right to

► Ask to see and get a copy of your health records

► Have corrections added to your health information

► Receive a notice that tells you how your health information may be used and shared

► Decide if you want to give your permission before your health information can be used or shared for certain purposes, such as for marketing

► Get a report on when and why your health information was shared for certain purposes

► If you believe your rights are being denied or your health information isn't being protected, you can

▷ File a complaint with your provider or health insurer

▷ File a complaint with the U.S. Government

You should get to know these important rights, which help you protect your health information. You can ask your provider or health insurer questions about your rights. You also can learn more about your rights, including how to file a complaint, from the website at www.hhs.gov/ocr/hipaa/ or by calling 1-866-627-7748; the phone call is free.

Page 1

Source: U.S. Department of Health and Human Services Office for Civil Rights

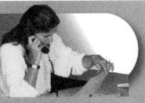

PRIVACY

The Law Sets Rules and Limits on Who Can Look At and Receive Your Information

For More Information

This is a brief summary of your rights and protections under the federal health information privacy law. You can learn more about health information privacy and your rights in a fact sheet called *"Your Health Information Privacy Rights"*. You can get this from the website at www.hhs.gov/ocr/hipaa/. You can also call 1-866-627-7748; the phone call is free.

Other privacy rights

Another law provides additional privacy protections to patients of alcohol and drug treatment programs. For more information, go to the website at www.samhsa.gov.

To make sure that your information is protected in a way that does not interfere with your health care, your information can be used and shared

- ▶ For your treatment and care coordination
- ▶ To pay doctors and hospitals for your health care and help run their businesses
- ▶ With your family, relatives, friends or others you identify who are involved with your health care or your health care bills, unless you object
- ▶ To make sure doctors give good care and nursing homes are clean and safe
- ▶ To protect the public's health, such as by reporting when the flu is in your area
- ▶ To make required reports to the police, such as reporting gunshot wounds

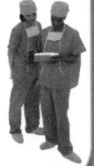

Your health information cannot be used or shared without your written permission unless this law allows it. For example, without your authorization, your provider generally cannot

- ▶ Give your information to your employer
- ▶ Use or share your information for marketing or advertising purposes
- ▶ Share private notes about your mental health counseling sessions

Published by:

U.S. Department of Health & Human Services Office for Civil Rights

The Law Protects the Privacy of Your Health Information

Providers and health insurers who are required to follow this law must keep your information private by

- ▶ Teaching the people who work for them how your information may and may not be used and shared
- ▶ Taking appropriate and reasonable steps to keep your health information secure

Page 2

189

Glossary of Terms and Important Concepts

Administrative law judge—The ALJ is the individual who will act on appeals at later stages.

Annual coordinated election period—In most cases, once people have enrolled in a Medicare drug plan, they will remain in that plan until the end of the plan year. They will be able to switch plans or disenroll during the Annual Coordinated Election Period (AEP), November 15—December 31 each year, with changes effective the following January 1. All people with Medicare can join, switch, or drop Medicare drug plans during the Annual Coordinated Election Period (AEP). The next AEP will be November 15 through December 31, 2006. Changes will be effective January 1, 2007.

Benefit period—A benefit period begins the first day you stay in a hospital or skilled nursing facility and ends when you have been out of the hospital or skilled nursing facility for 60 days in a row. If you go into the facility after one benefit period has ended, a new benefit period begins. There is no limit to the number of benefit periods you can have.

Brand name drug—These are prescription drugs for which there is not a generic option available. These drugs are still protected by patent and a generic substitute cannot be approved by the United States FDA until the patent period has expired.

Chronic care improvement program—These CCIPs are in select parts of the country and are designed to measure the impact of specialized services provided to at risk chronically ill seniors.

CMS—Centers for Medicare and Medicaid Services, the United States Federal Government Agency serving as the funding agency for Medicare Part D. Medicaid services are also provided through CMS.

Co-Payment—A required payment to obtain medications in the Medicare Part D Drug Program. This amount will vary depending upon whether the drug obtained is a generic or brand name product.

Coverage Gap—For most plans, the enrollee pays the first $250 of yearly drug costs, then 25% of the total drug costs between $250 and $2250, and 100% of costs between $2250 and $5100. After spending reaches a total of $5100 (or $3600 out of your pocket), catastrophic coverage begins and is the greater of $2 or $5 per prescription, or 5% coinsurance for each prescription. These amounts will change from year to year.

Creditable Coverage—This refers to prescription drug coverage that you may have from another insurance policy or from your current or former employer. Does this other coverage that you have meet or exceed the benefits offered through the Medicare Part D plans? Is it as good or better than the other drug coverage insurance that you have?

Deductible—The amount that must be paid by a participant before Medicare Part D coverage begins.

Donut Hole—The coverage gap that is present after initial coverage begins and ends and additional coverage starts. Between the coverage ending and restarting, the enrollee pays the entire cost of drugs for that period. Some of the prescription drug plans and Medicare Advantage programs will cover the partial costs of drugs in this interim. The trade-off is that the monthly premiums for the insurance coverage may be higher than otherwise.

Dual Eligibility—Persons who have both Medicare and Medicaid coverage are termed dual eligible. If you are dual eligible you will be automatically enrolled in a Medicare Part D prescription plan.

End Stage Renal Disease—If you are diagnosed with this kidney disease, end state renal disease, you are eligible for Medicare insurance coverage.

Fee for Service—Under the fee-for-service payment system, you can choose any licensed physician and use the services of any hospital, health care provider or facility certified by Medicare. Generally, a fee is paid each time a service is used. Medicare pays a share of your hospital, doctor, and other health care expenses. You are responsible for certain deductibles and coinsurance payments—the portion of the bill Medicare does not pay. You must also pay all permissible charges in excess of Medicare's approved amounts as well as charges for services not covered by Medicare. Some of those potential out-of-pocket costs can be avoided or reduced through the purchase of private insurance to supplement Medicare. It is called "Medigap" insurance and it is specifically designed to close some of the payment gaps in your Medicare coverage.

Food and Drug Administration—The FDA is the federal agency in the United States that monitors and approves the marketing, distribution, and use of prescription and over-the-counter medicines in the United States.

Formulary—A listing of drugs covered by a particular prescription drug plan in Medicare Part D. Coverage for specific drugs that you take may vary from plan to plan.

Generic drug—This is a less expensive version of a brand name drug. Generic drugs have received United States

Glossary

FDA approval prior to their being eligible for market entry. The brand name version of the same drug no longer has patent protection, or sole marketing privileges in the United States.

Health Maintenance Organization (HMO)—This is a combination insurance company and health services provider. Medicare Advantage plans in Medicare Part D may use HMOs to provide services to you.

Health Savings Account—A health savings account (HSA) is an account that you can put money into to save for future health and medical care expenses. There is a favorable tax situation available to you when you place funds in these accounts.

In-network Pharmacy—These are the pharmacies that can be used by you to obtain prescriptions with Medicare Part D coverage. Not all pharmacies are in the network of allowed pharmacies with each prescription drug plan or Medicare Advantage plan. You will need to check with your pharmacist to see if the pharmacy is a participant in the plan that you choose to sign up for.

Initial Enrollment Period—When you first become eligible for Medicare Part D services, you will have a seven (7) month period when you can sign up for coverage.

Low income subsidy—The LIS is an extra amount provided to you based upon your income and the number of members in your household. In general, if your income is less than 135% of the amount of the Federal Poverty Level you are eligible for this low income subsidy program.

Medication Therapy Management Services—These is as of yet undefined program to help seniors with individual specific programs to help them comply with their medications, and control their disease states.

Mail order pharmacy—A licensed pharmacy that serves patients by mailing prescriptions from the pharmacy to the individual's home.

Medicare Advantage—Formerly known as Medicare + Choice, it is now known as Medicare Advantage. This is the managed care option (Health Maintenance Organization [HMO] or Preferred Provider Organization [PPO]) providing extensive coverage. This segment of Medicare also includes coverage for prescription drugs. Individuals must sign up for Medicare Part C insurance. There is a premium payment required for participating in Medicare Advantage insurance programs.

Medicare Appeals Council—The MAC will act upon appeals from the administrative law judge (ALJ).

Medicare Cost Plan—A Medicare Cost Plan is a type of HMO. In a Medicare Cost Plan, if you get services outside of the plan's network without a referral, your Medicare-covered services will be paid for under the Original Medicare plan.

Medicare Part A—Inpatient hospital services, skilled nursing facilities, home care. Individuals are automatically enrolled as they reach the age of 65 years. There is not a premium payment required for obtaining Medicare Part A. This is financed by payroll taxes individuals pay. Other individuals may be eligible for Medicare health benefits at a younger age.

Medicare Part B—Supplemental Medical Insurance that pays for physician and other health care provider office visits, outpatient services, drugs administered in an outpatient clinic. Individuals must sign up for Medicare Part B insurance. This is an insurance component that does require that you pay a monthly premium.

Medicare Part C—Formerly known as Medicare + Choice, it is also known as Medicare Advantage. This is the managed care option (Health Maintenance Organization [HMO]) providing extensive coverage. This segment of Medicare also includes coverage for prescription drugs. Individuals must sign up for Medicare Part C insurance.

Glossary

195

There is a premium payment required for participating in Medicare Advantage insurance programs.

Medicare Part D—Prescription drug coverage under Medicare. Covers prescription drugs obtained from a community pharmacy or an outpatient hospital pharmacy. Individuals must sign up for Medicare Part D insurance. There is a premium payment required for participation in Medicare Part D insurance plans.

Medigap insurance. These are insurance plans that pay some of the expenses that Medicare will not pay for. These in the past have included prescription drug insurance plans.

Multiple drug tiers—Multiple drug tiers are part of the formulary system of prescription drug plans. You will pay differing amounts of co-payments for various types of drugs. These drugs are generic drugs, brand name drugs, and preferred drugs. Generic substitutes are drugs available (less expensively) than brand name drugs. Generics are available after the patent protection period runs out for brand name drugs. Brand name drugs are still protected by patents and do not have a generic substitute legally available. Preferred drugs are drugs that the prescription drug plan has negotiated for a lower price than normal with the manufacturer of the drug. It may be a brand name drug, but the price is lower than you would normally pay for it.

Non-formulary drug—Non-formulary drugs are drugs that the drug plan does not include in the drugs available to you as a plan member in the Medicare Part D program. You and your physician can petition the drug plan to have the drug covered. If you are successful in your petition, you will have coverage for this drug for the balance of the year. You have to repeat this process every year. If the petition is denied, there is an appeal process that you can follow to have the prescription drug plan review the decision to deny your petition.

Office of Inspector General—This department of the federal government evaluates providers of services and plans offered by companies and providers to beneficiaries. This office evaluates fraud, fraudulent claims, and issues fraud alerts to you as a Medicare recipient.

Ombudsman—Medicare has instituted an appointment of a Medicare Beneficiary Ombudsman to ensure people with Medicare get the information and help they need to understand their Medicare options, including their rights and protections. The Office of the Medicare Beneficiary Ombudsman will address processes for complaints and information request.

Out-of-network pharmacies. These are the pharmacies that are **not** part of the network of pharmacies used by prescription drug plans and Medicare Advantage plans that allow enrollees to obtain prescription medications.

Out-of-pocket expenses—These are the required amounts that you will have to pay in the Medicare Part D program until your deductible has been met, depending upon the plan chosen, these amounts may be small or large.

Patient assistance programs—These are the programs offered by various drug manufactures to provide you with reduced prices or free medications from the drugs that they manufacture. These plans will require you to sign up for coverage and provide statements of your income to check for eligibility. These programs are allowed to provide drugs to you as a Medicare Part D recipient. The drugs that are provided must fall outside of the drugs and payments provided through Medicare Part D.

Penalty—An additional continuing amount added to your monthly premium for Medicare Part B or for a Medicare prescription drug plan if you do not join when you are first eligible. You pay this amount as long as you have Medicare. There are some exceptions. For instance, you will not pay a penalty if you have creditable prescription drug coverage and do not enroll in a prescription drug when you are eligible to do so. If through no fault of your own your coverage is discontinued, you are not assessed this additional penalty when you do sign up for coverage.

Personal health information—PHI is information specifically about your health and health conditions. This is personal and private information that is protected by law. Please see Appendix F for details, your rights, what is involved, and what is expected of those providing care to you.

Petition—This is what must be done if you would like to challenge the formulary coverage of the particular prescription drug plan that you chose. Your physician can also petition to have a certain drug added to the formulary for a particular plan.

Pharmacy Network—The pharmacy network is the listing of pharmacies that you can use to obtain prescriptions from with your particular prescription drug plan. This network will vary from one part of the country to another. Also, there are some pharmacies that are national providers and can participate in plans anywhere. Please do not assume that your current pharmacy will be a participant in the pharmacy network for your prescription drug plan. You should verify this before you sign up for a particular plan if this is an important issue for you.

Preferred drug—Preferred drugs are drugs that the prescription drug plan has negotiated for a lower price than normal with the manufacturer of the drug. It may be a brand name drug, but the price is lower than you would normally pay for it.

Preferred provider organization—PPOs are providers in Medicare Advantage programs. It is a form of HMO that requires that you to select from a defined number of physicians, pharmacists, and hospitals from which to obtain care.

Prescription Drug Plan—These PDPs are the plans throughout the United States that will provide the insurance plan for which you sign up. Some of these plans are regional plans and some are national plans. Be sure to find out the coverage options for your particular prescription drug plan before you finalize signing up for the plan coverage.

Prior approval—Prior approval (PA) may be required with your particular prescription drug plan before one or more of your prescription medications may be filled and dispensed to you. This process of obtaining prior approval is processed by your pharmacy through consultation with your doctor. These services are provided by your pharmacy.

Prior authorization—Prior approval (PA) may be required with your particular prescription drug plan before one or more of your prescription medications may be filled and dispensed to you. This process of obtaining prior approval is processed by your pharmacy through consultation with your doctor. These services are provided by your pharmacy.

Quantity limits—These are limits placed on the days' supply of prescription medications that you can obtain in Medicare Part D prescription drug plans. Mail order pharmacies can provide a 90 day supply of medications. You can petition to have similar limits available to you in community pharmacies where you obtain your prescription drugs.

State Health Insurance Assistance Program. SHIPS are state helping agencies that have provided help with Medicare Part D questions, dilemmas, problems for thousands of Medicare recipients.

Step therapy—This is a requirement specified by some prescription plans. In step therapies you are required to try a less expensive medication to see if it works for you. If it does not then you can obtain a newer drug that your physician has prescribed for you. You and your physician can petition to allow you to directly obtain a prescribed drug without using a step therapy drug.

Supplemental Security Income—SSI is a Federal income supplement program funded by general tax revenues (not Social Security taxes): it is designed to help aged, blind, and disabled people, who have little or no income; and it provides cash to meet basic needs for food, clothing, and shelter.

Special enrollment periods—Special enrollment periods (SEP) are provided to individuals to sign up for coverage or switch coverage plans due to special circumstances. For example, Hurricane Katrina evacuees have been granted SEPs due to their specific circumstances. Medicare beneficiaries who qualify for the Low Income Subsidy (LIS) were able to sign up for it and choose and join a prescription drug plan after the May 15, 2006, deadline. Special Enrollment Periods (SEPs) will also apply to individuals who are enrolled into a drug plan by a State Pharmaceutical Assistance Program. You may switch drug plans once by the end of 2006.

Tiered Cop-payments. Multiple drug tiers are part of the formulary system of prescription drug plans. You will pay differing amounts of co-payments for various types of drugs depending upon which tier the drug is from. These drugs are generic drugs, brand name drugs, and preferred drugs. Generic substitutes are drugs available (less expensively) than a brand name drugs. Generics are available after the patent protection period runs out for brand name drugs. Brand name drugs are still protected by patents and do not have a generic substitute legally available. Preferred drugs are drugs that the prescription drug plan has negotiated for a lower price than normal with the manufacturer of the drug. It may be a brand name drug, but the price is lower than you would normally pay for it.

Transition period—The transition period is the time between your signing up for a Medicare Part D Plan and the time when your benefits begin. The prescription drug plans are required to allow you to continue on your current drug regimens and have coverage for a 30 day period. If you are in a long-term care facility (nursing home) you are allowed a 180 day grace period. These periods are in place to allow your physician and you to select a drug that is covered under the prescription drug plan formulary.

True out of pocket (TrOOP) spending—These are the calculated amounts of spending by you during the year that count toward you reaching other coverage amounts in the Medicare Part D program. Medicare Part D Plans will calculate this amount for members in their plans.

Veterans Administration—The VA provides care for war veterans eligible for services.